Q&A Color Review of

General Critical Care

H. Mathilda Horst
MD, FACS, FCCM
Henry Ford Hospital
Detroit, Michigan, USA

Riyad C. Karmy-Jones
MD, FRCSC, FRCSC (CT), FACS, FCCP
University of Washington
Seattle, Washington, USA

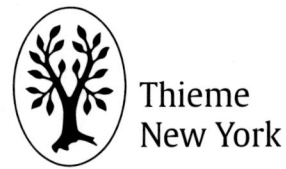

Thieme
New York

Preface

The management of patients in a critical care setting requires a subtle integration of applied and theoretical physiology; clinical judgement and understanding of outcomes and outcomes-based medicine; a basic understanding of medical engineering; and, most importantly, dotting the i's and crossing the t's, in other words, attention to small details. Patients in the ICU tend to get categorized into flow sheets and it is easy to forget that the care of patients involves evolution of the disease process over a period of time rather than in snippets of time. Attention to minor details is at times exhausting and may even be distracting, but this is probably the most important aspect of intensive care. Some physicians use physiological formulas in understanding the basic science and review collected data as the predominant basis of their management, whereas others use sound clinical judgement and instinct. Both general approaches are valid, but an understanding of both approaches is essential to make rational decisions in the care of patients.

This title is designed to serve as both a review book and as a reference manual. The goals of the book are to bring out different aspects of critical care management and to allow the reader to understand the science and Gestalt of critical care medicine. For instance, using a pulmonary artery occlusion catheter to determine the effectiveness of therapy requires an understanding of the controversies surrounding its appropriateness, as well as an understanding of how the catheter actually works in certain settings.

The questions were supplied by an international group of authors and the different approaches cover both written and oral examinations. It is hoped that these questions may also serve as examples of questions that can be used on teaching rounds for medical students and residents. The questions are based on years of experience in both surgical and medical intensive care. We would like to thank the residents and nurses whose excellent care and quest for knowledge has stimulated the authors to contribute to this book.

First published in the United States of America in 2003 by:
Thieme New York, 333 Seventh Avenue
New York, NY 10001, USA

ISBN 1–58890–155–6

Library of Congress Cataloging-in-Publication Data
is available from the publisher

This book, including all parts thereof, is legally protected by copyright. Any use, exploitation, or commercialization outside the narrow limits set by copyright legislation, without the publisher's consent, is illegal and liable to prosecution. This applies in particular to photostat reproduction, copying, mimeographing or duplication of any kind, translating, preparation of microfilms, and electronic data processing and storage.

Important note: Medical knowledge is ever-changing. As new research and clinical experience broaden our knowledge, changes in treatment and drug therapy may be required. The authors and editors of the material herein have consulted sources believed to be reliable in their efforts to provide information that is complete and in accord with the standards accepted at the time of publication. However, in view of the possibility of human error by the authors, editors, or publisher of the work herein, or changes in medical knowledge, neither the authors, editors, or publisher, nor any other party who has been involved in the preparation of this work, warrants that the information contained herein is in every respect accurate or complete, and they are not responsible for any errors or omissions or for the results obtained from use of such information. Readers are encouraged to confirm the information contained herein with other sources. For example, readers are advised to check the product information sheet included in the package of each drug they plan to administer to be certain that the information contained in this publication is accurate and that changes have not been made in the recommended dose or in the contraindications for administration. This recommendation is of particular importance in connection with new or infrequently used drugs.

Some of the product names, patents, and registered designs referred to in this book are in fact registered trademarks or proprietary names even though specific reference to this fact is not always made in the text. Therefore, the appearance of a name without designation as proprietary is not to be construed as a representation by the publisher that it is in the public domain.

Copyright © 2003 Manson Publishing Ltd, 73 Corringham Road, London NW11 7DL, UK

Printed in Spain

Contributors

Keith J. Anderson, BSc (Hons), MB, ChB, FRCA
Nuffield Department of Anaesthetics, Oxford, UK

Tamir Ben-Menachim, MD, MS
Henry Ford Hospital, Detroit, Michigan, USA

Susan Brundage, MD
Ben Taub General Hospital, Houston, Texas, USA

Gretchen Carter
University of Michigan, Grosse Pointe, Michigan, USA

Yvonne Carter, MD
University of Washington, Seattle, Washington, USA

Barry A. Finegan, MB, ChB, FRCPC, FRARCSI
University of Alberta, Edmonton, Alberta, Canada

Glendon M. Gardner, MD
Henry Ford Hospital, Detroit, Michigan, USA

Magnus A. Garrioch, MB, ChB, FRCA
Southern General Hospital and University of Glasgow, Glasgow, UK

Mario Gasparri, MD
Medical College of Wisconsin, Milwaukee, Wisconsin, USA

Stavros Georganos, MD
Henry Ford Hospital, Detroit, Michigan, USA

Benjamin Guslits, MD, MBA, FRCPC
University Hospital, Michigan, USA

Andrew Hamilton, MD, FRCSC, FRCSC (CT)
University of Manitoba, Winnipeg, Manitoba, USA

H. Mathilda Horst, MD, FACS, FCCM
Henry Ford Hospital, Detroit, Michigan, USA

Troy P. Houseworth, MD
Case Western Reserve University/Henry Ford Hospital, Detroit, Michigan, USA

James Jeng, MD, FACS
Washington Hospital Center, Washington, DC, USA

Major Donald Jenkins, MD USAF
Lacklund Airforce Base, Texas, USA

Jay Johannigman, MD, FACS
University Hospital
Cincinnati, Ohio, USA

Riyad C. Karmy-Jones, MD, FRCS, FRCS (CT), FACS, FCCP
University of Washington, Seattle, Washington, USA

David P. Kissinger, MD, FACS
Lackland Air Force Base, San Antonio, Texas, USA

Kurt A. Kralovich, MD
Henry Ford Hospital, Detroit, Michigan, USA

Daniel A. Ladin, MD, FACS
Kaiser Medical Group, Clackamas, Oregon, USA

Gordon Lees, MD, FRCSC
University of Alberta, Edmonton, Alberta, Canada

Joseph W. Lewis, Jr, MD
Henry Ford Hospital, Detroit, Michigan, USA

Catherine LeGalley, MD
West Bloomfield, Michigan, USA

Cairan J. McNamee, MD, MSc, FRCSC
University of Alberta, Edmonton, Alberta, Canada

Contributors

Daniel C. Morris, MD, ABEM
Henry Ford Hospital, Detroit, Michigan, USA

Nutritional Support Team
Henry Ford Hospital, Detroit, Michigan, USA

Farouck N. Obeid, MD, FACS
Henry Ford Hospital, Detroit, Michigan, USA

Brant Oelschlager, MD
University of Washington, Seattle,
Washington, USA

Kevin J. O'Hare, MB, ChB, FRCA
Southern General Hospital, Glasgow, UK

Amy Pinney, MD
University of Toledo, Toledo, Ohio, USA

Iraklis I. Pipinos, MD
Henry Ford Hospital, Detroit, Michigan, USA

Stewart Pringle, MB, ChB, MRCGP, MRCOG
Southern General Hospital, Glasgow, UK

Ian Ramsay, MB, ChB, MRCOG
Southern General Hospital, Glasgow, UK

Mark Ratch, EMT-P
Edmonton Fire Department, Edmonton, Alberta, Canada

Ilan S. Rubinfeld, MD
University of California at San Diego, California, USA

Marc J. Shapiro, MD
St Louis University, St Louis, Missouri, USA

Alexander D. Shephard, MD, FACS
Henry Ford Hospital, Detroit, Michigan, USA

Harald Schoeppner, MD, FACP
Tacoma General Hospital, Tacoma, Washington, USA

Victor Sorenson, MD, FACS
Henry Ford Hospital, Detroit, Michigan, USA

John Spiers, MD
Hotel D'ieu Grace Hospital, Windsor, Ontario, Canada

Lorie Thomas, PhD
University of Washington, Seattle, Washington, USA

Eric Vallières, MD, FRCS
University of Washington, Seattle, Washington, USA

Vic Velanovic, MD, FACS
Henry Ford Hospital, Detroit, Michigan, USA

Mary H. van Wijngaarden, MD, FRCSC
University of Alberta Hospitals, Edmonton, Alberta, Canada

James W. Wagner, MD
Henry Ford Hospital, Detroit, Michigan, USA

Ira S. Wollner, MD, FACP
Henry Ford Hospital, Detroit, Michigan, USA

Douglas E. Wood, MD, FACS, FCCP
University of Washington, Seattle, Washington, USA

Janice L. Zimmerman, MD, FCCM
Ben Taub General Hospital, Houston, Texas, USA

Dedications
For Judith (H.M.H.)
For Don and Linda (R.K.J.)

1–3: Questions

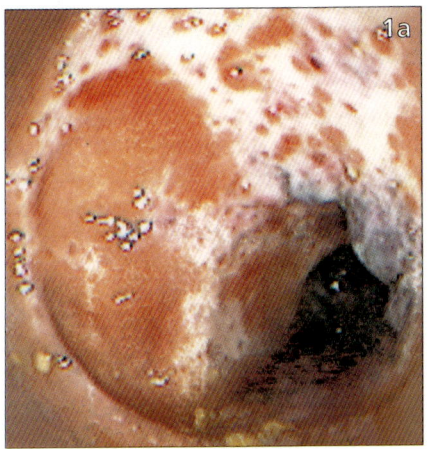
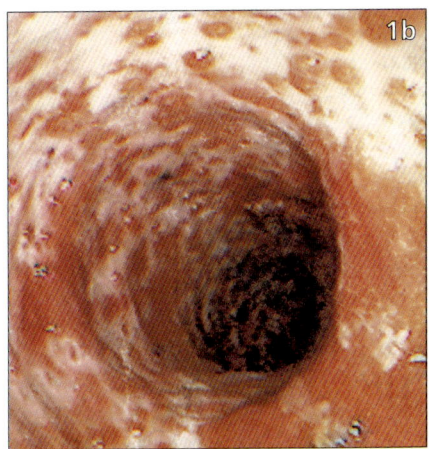

1 A 66-year-old male is admitted to the coronary care unit because of exacerbation of his CHF. He develops crampy abdominal pain and passes blood-tinged diarrhea. Physical examination reveals only a mild abdominal tenderness and plain films demonstrate only ileus. A colonoscopy is performed and reveals the findings shown (**1a, b**). What is the diagnosis? What is the management?

2 A 15-year-old female with a known history of depression and suicide gestures presents to the emergency department after having an argument with her parents. The patient says that she took several handfuls of acetaminophen (paracetamol) approximately 2 hours ago. What is the minimum toxic dose of of this drug in children?
A 100 mg/kg.
B 120 mg/kg.
C 140 mg/kg.
D 160 mg/kg.

3 A 17-year-old male underwent repair of a rotator cuff injury under general anesthesia. The surgical repair is uneventful, but as the incision is being closed, the patient's end-tidal CO_2 tension and body temperature begin to rise. A diagnosis of malignant hyperthermia is made. Inhalation anesthesia is discontinued and the patient is treated with intravenous fluids, hyperventilation on 100% oxygen, cooling, and given 5 mg/kg dantrolene, before his condition stabilizes.
   The patient is transferred to the ICU for continued monitoring. Which of the following complications may be associated with the development or treatment of malignant hyperthermia?
A Ventricular dysrhythmias.
B Acute renal failure.
C Recurrence of malignant hyperthermia.
D Disseminated intravascular coagulation.

1–3: Answers

1 This is a typical endoscopic picture of ischemic colitis. Colonoscopy is the best method of making the diagnosis, as plain films and CT scans, in the absence of frank gangrene, are usually nonspecific. Ischemic colitis is classified as either nongangrenous (85%) or gangrenous (15%). Nongangrenous, in turn, is divided into acute, reversible (60–70%) or chronic, nonreversible. Etiologies are multifactorial but all relate to decreased mucosal flow. Surgical management is required acutely if there is ongoing sepsis, evidence of peritonitis, free air noted on radiographs, gangrene noted endoscopically and, or, persistent bleeding or protein-losing colonopathy lasting for more than 14 days. In this case, attention would be directed at improving the CHF, avoiding vasopressors and digoxin, and careful monitoring. Treatment in other cases is usually supportive, and includes nasogastric decompression, parenteral nutrition, avoiding enemas, and optimizing blood flow.

2 C. Acetaminophen (paracetamol) is found in hundreds of prescription and nonprescription medications. Because of its widespread availability, both accidental and intentional overdoses are common. Acetaminophen is metabolized in the liver via glucuronide and sulfate conjugation. In overdose situations, these pathways are saturated and acetaminophen is metabolized by the cytochrome P450 system via glutathione conjugation. This pathway produces a toxic intermediate metabolite which is responsible for hepatic damage and cell death. Clinical manifestations of toxicity can be subtle, nonspecific, and may not manifest until 24–36 hours after ingestion. Signs and symptoms include anorexia, nausea and vomiting, right upper quadrant tenderness, and jaundice. The minimum toxic dose in children is 140 mg/kg and in adults >7.5 g. The Rumack–Matthew nomogram can be used as a guide to predict hepatic toxicity. Treatment involves administration of N-acetylcysteine. Outcomes of acetaminophen ingestion can range from complete recovery to fulminant hepatic failure. Liver function test elevations do not necessarily correlate with clinical outcome.

3 All of the above. Malignant hyperthermia is a disease associated with abnormal calcium flux and accelerated metabolism of skeletal muscle. The prolonged muscle contracture leads to excessive heat production as well as myocyte necrosis. Hyperkalemia develops as a result of cell necrosis and metabolic acidosis. In severe cases, ventricular dysrhythmias, including ventricular fibrillation, may occur. Rhabdomyolysis releases toxic metabolites such as myoglobin and free radicals into the circulation. Acute tubular necrosis may result. Disseminated intravascular coagulation is a frequent occurrence in fulminant malignant hyperthermia. It is thought to be related to the release of thromboplastins secondary to the shock state and to the release of cellular contents following membrane destruction. Despite initial treatment with dantrolene, malignant hyperthermia may recur during the immediate or late postoperative period. Patients, therefore, require close monitoring in an intensive care environment for acute recurrence.

4–7: Questions

4 A 65-year-old female presents to the emergency department with progressive dyspnea over 3 days associated with fever and chills. Vital signs are: HR 96/min, BP 137/84 mmHg (18.3/11.2 kPa), RR 32/min and temperature 39.2°C (102.5°F). Evaluation revealed an elderly female in respiratory distress with both inspiratory and expiratory stridor. The pharynx is edematous and an erythematous lesion is noted over her neck and upper thorax (4).

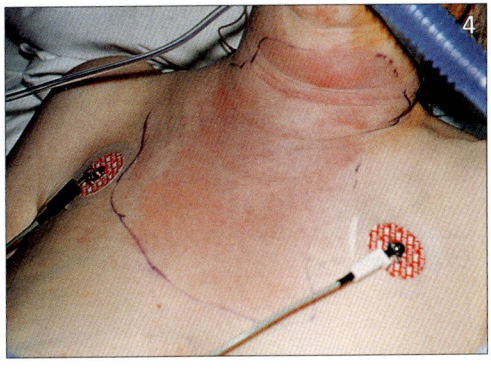

Appropriate management of this patient would include which of the following:
A Induction of general anesthesia followed by orotracheal intubation.
B Blind nasotracheal intubation.
C Tracheostomy under general anesthesia.
D Maintaining spontaneous ventilation and performance of a fiberoptic intubation.
E No intervention at this time. Admit to the ICU for observation and antibiotic therapy.

5 A 50-year-old male is in the ICU after undergoing colostomy, sigmoid resection, and Hartman's pouch procedures for a perforated diverticulitis. His vital signs are: BP 110/60 mmHg (14.7/8.0 kPa), HR 100/min, RR 18/min. On the ventilator his tidal volume is 700 ml, FiO_2 90%, and PEEP 15 cm/H_2O. Barometric pressure is 760 mmHg (101.3 kPa). His laboratory findings are given below:

Hemoglobin	1 g/l (0.1 g/dl)	WBC 16 x 10⁹/l (16,000/mm³)
	ABG	Mixed venous gas
PO_2	60 mmHg (8.0 kPa)	35 mmHg (4.7 kPa)
PCO_2	31 mmHg (4.1 kPa)	34 mmHg (4.5 kPa)
pH	7.4	7.42
SaO_2 sat	91%	64%

What is the $AVDO_2$?

6 List the five main causes of a difficult intubation in the ICU.

7 Which organism is a cause of 'atypical' pneumonia. It is weakly Gram-negative and requires increased amounts of iron and cysteine for growth in culture.

4–7: Answers

4 D. This patient had erysipelas, associated with upper airway compromise. When airway compromise is imminent, expectant management with observation in the ICU may lead to disastrous results. The preferential way to manage such an airway is to secure it by maintaining spontaneous ventilation and intubating the patient under direct vision with a fiberoptic bronchoscope. This affords the operator the opportunity to examine the airway and position the endotracheal tube below any tracheal lesion. Blind nasal intubation is not advised when pharyngeal edema is present as the trauma of manipulating the endotracheal tube in the pharynx may exacerbate the pre-existing pathology. Patients with impending airway collapse should not receive general anesthesia as this may precipitate complete airway occlusion with inability to ventilate the patient by bag-valve-mask. In all situations of upper airway compromise, a physician skilled in the performance of a tracheostomy or cricothyrotomy should be immediately available.

5 $AVDO_2$ is calculated by subtracting the mixed venous blood oxygen content from the arterial blood oxygen content:

$$AVDO_2 = CaO_2 - CvO2 \text{ where } CaO_2 - (Hgb \times 1.34 \times SaO_2) + (PaO_2 \times 0.003) \text{ and } CvO_2 = (Hgb \times 1.34 \times SvO_2) + (PvO_2 \times 0.003)$$

The content 1.34 is the number of milliliters of oxygen that can bind to a gram of hemoglobin (Hgb). The amount of unbound oxygen dissolved in the blood is represented by ($PO_2 \times 0.003$). The normal $AVDO_2$ is approximately 5% volume. A hypermetabolic state is present if the $AVDO_2$ is <5% volume. Any cause of a low cardiac output will elevate the oxygen content difference.

6 (1) *Obesity.* All obese patients must be considered difficult due to both anatomical factors and the difficulties of instrumentation of the airway. **(2)** *Prominent front teeth* (buck teeth). Prevents instrumentation of the oropharynx by failure to insert a laryngoscope. **(3)** *Decreased atlanto-occipital movement,* e.g. ankylosing spondylitis and rheumatoid arthritis. **(4)** *Receding mandible or micrognathia.* Both prevent insertion of the laryngoscope. **(5)** *A high arched palate* leads to relative override of the front teeth and consequent difficulties in placing an ET tube.

In addition other factors need to be remembered: swollen airways after trauma or maxillofacial surgery; the presence of a beard may conceal a receding mandible; any surgery on the neck, e.g. thyroidectomy or carotid surgery, may lead to a lower airway distortion and difficulty in intubation. *Do not embark on a rapid sequence induction in these patients.* Fiberoptic intubation or tracheostomy may be required (when the patient is awake).

7 *Legionella pneumophila.*

8–10: Questions

8 An otherwise healthy newborn male, weighing 2.4 kg (5 lb 5 oz) and born of an uneventful pregnancy and delivery, develops tachypnea at 48 hours of life. His SaO_2 is 90% in room air and 99% with 0.75 l/min of O_2. There is no evidence of congenital heart disease and an echocardiogram is normal. A chest X-ray was taken (**8**).

The optimal (long-term) management of this condition is which of the following?
A Trocarcannula decompression of the left chest.
B Selective endobronchial intubation.
C Rigid bronchoscopy to suction mucous plugs.
D ECMO.
E Thoracotomy and resection of the involved lobe/segment.

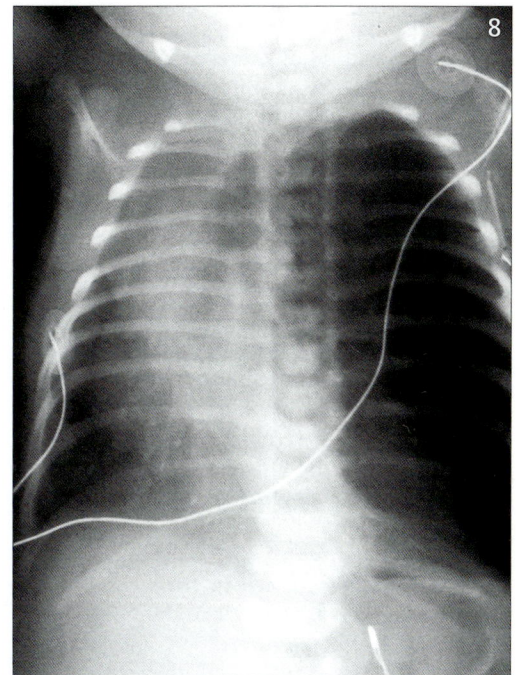

9 A radionuclide scan is undertaken after laparoscopic cholecystectomy (**9a, b**).
i. What does it demonstrate?
ii. What is the most appropriate next step?
A Exploratory laparotomy.
B A CT scan or ultrasound-guided aspiration of the fluid.
C Laparoscopic exploration.
D Endoscopic retrograde cholangiopancreatography and papillotomy.

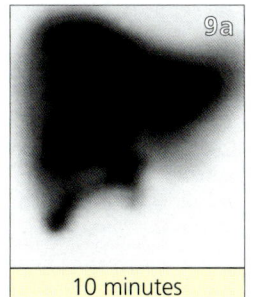
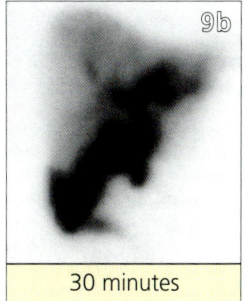

10 What is the MAC of an inhalational agent?

8–10: Answers

8 E. Congenital lobar emphysema is almost always present at birth, becomes rapidly progressive, and usually affects only one lobe, invariably the upper lobe, but in very rare instances may be bilateral. Associated anomalies are uncommon and with progressive distension of the affected lobe, there is mediastinal shift and atelectasis of the ipsilateral lower lobe and ultimately the contralateral lung. As a temporary measure, selective contralateral endobronchial intubation may be used but the definitive treatment is urgent thoracotomy and resection of the involved lobe/segment. The majority of children present within the first 4 weeks of life but occasionally the condition will not be diagnosed until later childhood.

9 i. The scan demonstrates extravasation of tracer from the biliary tree.
ii. D. The risk of biliary complication following laparoscopic cholecystectomy (0.5–5.0%) compares to an open cholecystectomy (0.1–1.0%). The most common complication is caused by incorrect placement of the cystic duct clips, or dislodgement of these clips during the operation. This leads to biliary leakage and eventual peritonitis. Other injuries include partial or complete common bile duct injury, inadvertent clipping of the common bile duct, and common bile duct strictures. Abdominal pain, jaundice and fever are clues to a biliary leak. The patient is best evaluated with either ultrasound to show a fluid collection, or radionuclide scan to demonstrate a leak from the biliary system. An endoscopic retrograde cholangiopancreatography can define the biliary anatomy as well as allowing the performance of a sphincterotomy and stent placement for drainage. For cystic duct stump leaks, this is usually all that is required for treatment. In patients with large bile collections or signs of peritonitis, transcutaneous drainage of the bile via ultrasound or CT scan guidance is helpful. In those patients found to have an obstructed duct, or who are septic, a laparotomy must then be performed and either primary repair of the common bile duct over T-tube or resection with choledochoenterostomy. Laparoscopy in the early postoperative period may be helpful, but often adhesions and edema make it difficult to define the anatomy.

10 The MAC of an agent, expressed as a percentage, is defined as the minimum alveolar concentration required to prevent reaction to a surgical stimulus (skin incision) in 50% of patients. It is measured in conditions of 100% oxygen and at atmospheric pressure. It correlates with the potency of an individual inhalational agent. The MAC value for halothane is 0.75% and for sevoflurane is 1.7%.

11–13: Questions

11 This 34-year-old male developed jaundice, increased abdominal pain, and vomited blood, 3 days after a road traffic accident. A CT scan (**11a, b**) was obtained. What is the diagnosis and management?

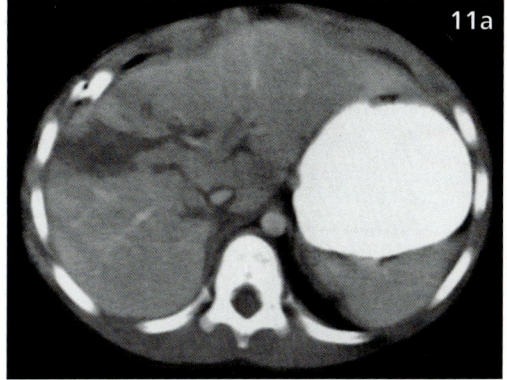

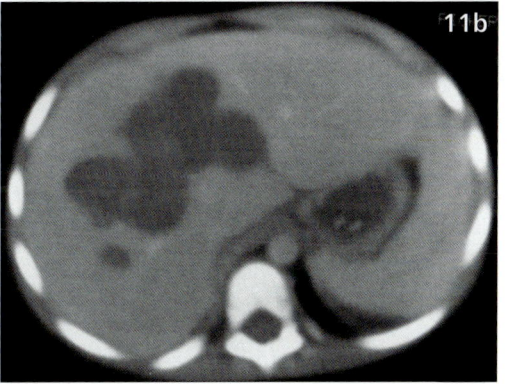

12 A typical capnography curve is shown (**12**). Label the four phases (I–IV). Describe what each phase represents and conditions that may alter the appearance of each phase.

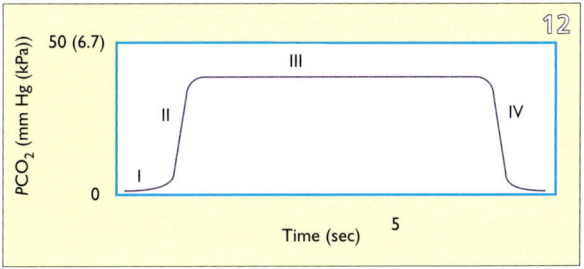

13 Discuss the relative merits of 'early' versus 'late' surgery for subarachnoid hemorrhage.

11–13: Answers

11 The CT scan shows a large central hematoma of the liver. The possibility of hematobilia should be considered. Other possibilities include a combined liver abscess or biliary disease with stress gastritis. An angiogram will be both therapeutic and diagnostic in this case.

12 *Phase I*: inspiratory baseline. CO_2 at this phase should be zero. Elevation of the inspiratory baseline indicates that CO_2 is being rebreathed. This may be the result of equipment failure. *Phase II*: the expiratory upstroke is steep. The prolonged upstroke indicates delay of movement of CO_2 from lungs to sampling site. This can be seen in patients with COPD or bronchospasm. *Phase III*: the expiratory plateau represents the V/Q continuum in the lung. The steepness of the plateau is directly related to the degree of airway resistance. Patients absent of any lung disease have a uniform expiratory plateau. Smokers or asthmatics have a steeper slope. A biphasic waveform occurs in patients who have extremely different individual lungs. This can occur with severe rotary kyphoscoliosis or be the result of mainstem bronchial intubation. Leaks in the sampling line cause an abnormally low expiratory plateau. *Phase IV*: the inspiratory downstroke is normally quite steep. A prolonged, slanted inspiratory downstroke is the result of a missing or incompetent inspiratory valve.

13 Early surgery usually implies within 0–3 days, late 11–14 days. The benefits of early surgery are that it prevents rebleeding and permits hypervolemic-hypertensive therapy. Late surgery is technically easier and there is reduced chance of intraoperative aneurysmal rupture. The decision is affected by clinical presentation and technical aspects. Clinical presentation can be graded by the Hunt and Hess scale. *Grade 1*: alert with minimal headache. *Grade 2*: alert with moderate headache (cranial nerve palsy allowed). *Grade 3*: lethargic or confused, or with mild focal defect. *Grade 4*: stuporous, moderate to severe hemiparesis, with possible early decerebrate rigidity. *Grade 5*: deep coma, decerebrate rigidity, and moribund appearance.

It will be apparent that to a certain extent this grading system is subjective. Early surgery in grades 1–2 appears to be associated with better outcomes. Early surgery (within 24 hours) and 'triple-H' therapy is the best approach with grades 1–3 presentation. Whether or not grades 4–5 should be approached by this is not clear.

Wide based and posterior circulating aneurysms are more technically challenging and may be better managed by late surgery.

14, 15: Questions

14 What is the difference between incidence and prevalence? Why is this difference important?

15 A 28-year-old homosexual male presents with a progressive skin rash over most of his body for 3 weeks and the development 4 days before presentation of bilateral swollen, painful knees. His vital signs were: BP 112/175 mmHg (15.0/23.3 kPa), HR 105/min, RR 22/min, temperature 39.8°C (103.7°F). Skin examination revealed generalized erythematous papules and plaques with scale, and severe fissuring of the scalp, palms, and soles (**15a**). Bilateral prominent knee effusions were noted (**15b**). The mucous membranes and conjunctivae were not involved.
i. What should be considered in the differential diagnosis of the skin lesions?
ii. What other information should be sought in the history?

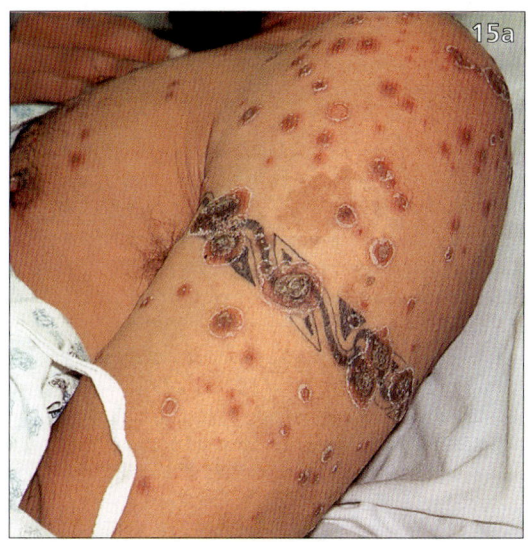

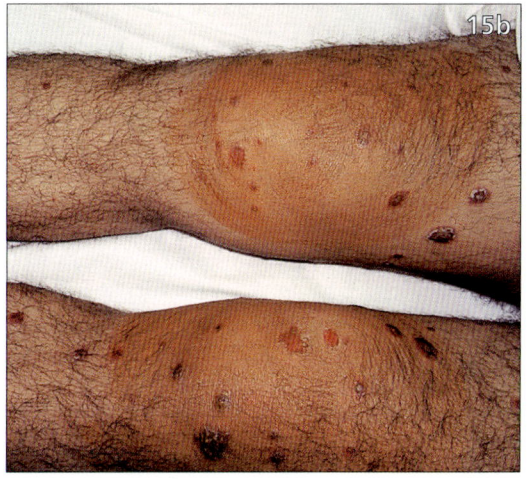

13

14, 15: Answers

14 Incidence is defined as the number of new cases occurring per given population over the course of a given time period. Typically it is given as:

incidence = number of new cases/100,000 people/year.

In a critical care setting, the units used to described the incidence of nosocomial infections may be number of new cases/100 patients/30 days. Prevalence is defined as the number of existing cases per given population. Typically it is given as:

prevalence = number of existing cases/100,000 people.

Note specifically there is no time frame, unlike incidence. Prevalence and incidence measure two different epidemiological facts. These measures may or may not be related. For example, in the early 1980s, the incidence of AIDS was increasing from year to year, although the overall prevalence of the disease was quite low. This was primarily due to ignorance of its spread and the short life expectancy of AIDS patients. In recent years, the incidence has decreased dramatically, primarily through education on how it is spread, but the prevalence has increased dramatically, primarily due to patients living longer with the disease. From the standpoint of diagnosis, prevalence is more important that incidence. The prevalence of a disease affects the reliability of a test. Basically, the higher the prevalence of a disease, the more likely that a positive test result reflects a true positive and a negative result reflects a false negative. Conversely, the lower the prevalence, the more likely that a negative test result reflects a true negative and a positive test result a false positive.

15 i. Papulosquamous disorders should be considered in the differential diagnosis of these skin lesions. Notably, this patient has evidence of systemic involvement with fever and knee effusions. Although erythema multiforme and Stevens–Johnson syndrome often present with severe systemic toxicity, the scaling and fissuring is not characteristic of these disorders. The appearance of the lesions does not suggest a primary skin infection, such as cellulitis and impetigo. Possible etiologies of these erythematous, scaling lesions include secondary syphilis, tinea corporis, seborrheic dermatitis, and psoriasis. This patient actually has generalized psoriasis.
ii. Sudden onset of previously undiagnosed psoriasis or acute worsening of pre-existing disease may indicate HIV infection. Psoriasis may be the initial sign of HIV infection and is generally considered to be a poor prognostic indicator. Information concerning risk factors for HIV transmission and symptoms such as weight loss, chronic diarrhea, or other infections should be sought. On further questioning, this patient admitted to intermittent diarrhea for 1 month and unprotected sexual practices. The tattoos were done by a friend and also could potentially serve as a source of HIV transmission. Serology for HIV in this patient was positive.

16–18: Questions

16 With regard to **15**, what further examinations are indicated?

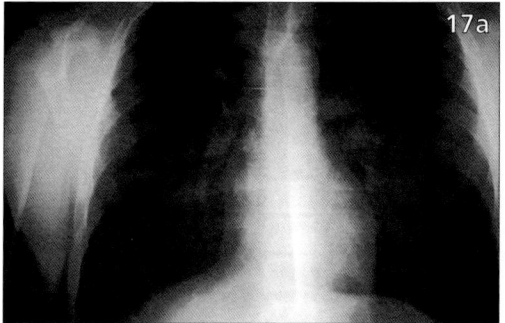
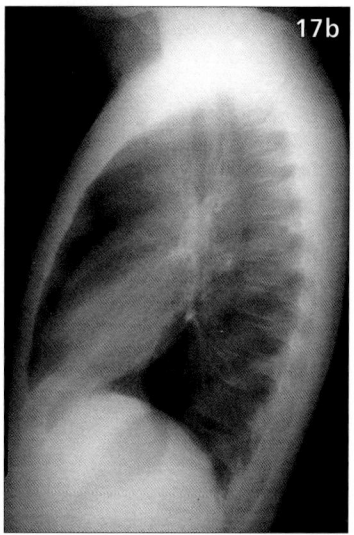

17 A 14-year-old male presented with a cough, wheeze, and mild chest pain after shooting pins through a home made blowgun. He had added a portion of a shoelace to the back of the pin to act as a tail. While shooting them, he inadvertently inhaled one of the pins. A chest X-ray is taken (**17a, b**). The best approach is:
A Antibiotics and observation.
B Removal in the emergency room with a fiberoptic scope.
C Removal in the operating room with a fiberoptic scope.
D Removal in the operating room with a rigid bronchoscope.

18 This piece of equipment is normally attached to the end of the expiratory limb of a breathing system (**18**).
i. What is it?
ii. How does application of this piece of equipment improve oxygenation?

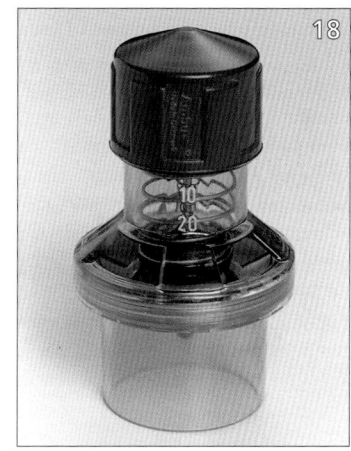

16–18: Answers

16 Certainly, HIV testing and a rapid plasma reagin (RPR) should be obtained. In addition, arthrocentesis of the knee effusions should be performed to rule out septic arthritis. The characteristics of this patient's joint fluid were WBC 9.5×10^9/l (9.5×10^3/mm^3) with 52% polymorphonuclear leukocytes and 43% lymphocytes, RBC 225 mm^3, glucose 3.22 mmol/l (58 mg/dl), and protein 44 g/l (4.4 g/dl). In this case, the results are most compatible with an inflammatory arthropathy secondary to psoriasis rather than bacterial infection. Arthritis occurs in approximately 30% of HIV-infected persons with psoriasis.

Treatment for this patient included hospital admission due to his inability to walk and care for himself as well as to rule out serious coinfection as a cause of fever. He was treated with antibiotics for secondary local infection from the skin lesions. Treatment for the psoriasis included topical steroids and medications for pruritus. Systemic steroids were not initiated due to the concerns of other infections and worsening immunosuppression.

17 D. Flexible endoscopy can be an easy outpatient diagnostic procedure but when an impacted foreign object is noted, rigid endoscopy in the operating room is generally felt to be safer by thoracic surgeons. Acute onset of cough and 'asthma' should suggest a central airway process, including aspira-

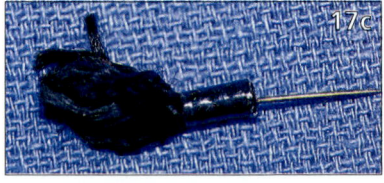

tion of foreign body. In this case the pin (17c), with wrapped shoe string, was impacted in the right upper lung bronchus with the tip imbedded in the medial main stem bronchus. It was removed using a rigid bronchoscope by grasping the pin, advancing it back into the right upper lung and then pulling it out point first.

18 The piece of equipment illustrated is a PEEP valve. It is attached to the expiratory limb of an Ambu bag or other temporary ventilation circuitry when the maintenance of PEEP is essential to prevent de-oxygenation. PEEP is applied to the lungs under conditions of atalectasis or other reasons of reduced functional residual capacity, e.g. ARDS, to attempt to open alveoli that are not participating in gas exchange. The ventilation perfusion ratio within the lung improves with a concurrent increase in the patient's oxygenation.

ii. The application of a small amount of PEEP to ventilated patients, i.e. 2–3 cmH$_2$O, is always helpful as the human larynx usually provides this amount of end-expiratory pressure in healthy subjects. Although this is good practice when setting a ventilator, it is not usually necessary for short-term ventilation when a PEEP valve such as that illustrated is being used. This PEEP valve should only be used when higher levels of PEEP are considered essential. It is to be noted that there are graded marks along the side of the apparatus to indicate how much PEEP is being applied. The maximum that can be applied using this device is 20 cmH$_2$O. This could be whilst transferring a patient on a temporary or portable ventilator, or when using an Ambu bag for short-term bedside ventilation when changing a ventilator on a patient who is 'PEEP dependent'.

19–21: Questions

19 Match one of the the electrolyte profiles A–E in the table with the following patient: a 20-year-old male with type I diabetes mellitus, gastric obstruction, severe vomiting, who stopped insulin 3 days ago.

	Na+ [1]	K+ [1]	Cl- [1]	HCO$_3^-$ [1]	Creatinine [2]	PCO$_2$ [3]	pH
A	140	3.7	95	33	106 (1.2)	65 (8.7)	7.33
B	135	4.7	86	24	168 (1.9)	40 (5.3)	7.40
C	143	3.1	88	41	133 (1.5)	65 (8.7)	7.42
D	137	4.0	102	15	115 (1.3)	30 (4.0)	7.33
E	140	4.0	105	10	88 (1.0)	17 (2.3)	7.39

[1] mmol/l, mEq/l   [2] μmol/l (mg/dl)   [3] mmHg (kPa)

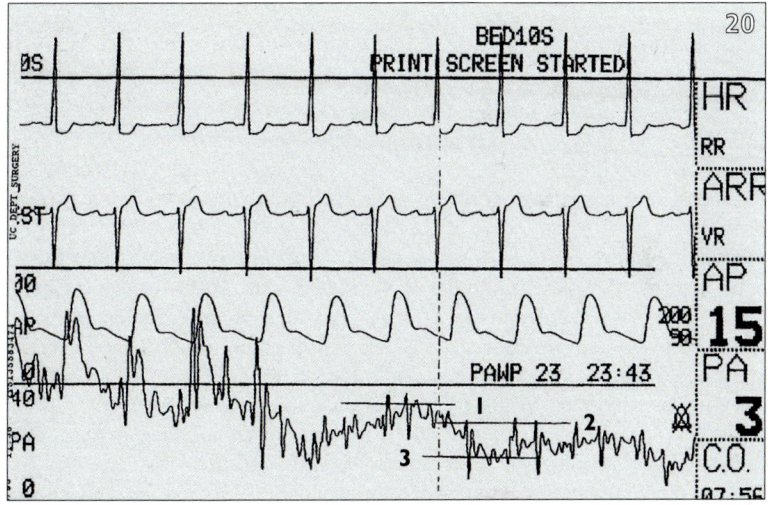

20 The illustration (20) depicts a tracing from a Swann–Ganz catheter during estimation of wedge pressure. The patient is intubated on the pressure-controlled ventilation mode and is not breathing spontaneously. Is the correct estimation of wedge pressure at point 1, 2, or 3?

21 What are the most common drugs and solutions known to cause anaphylaxis or anaphylactic reactions?

19–21: Answers

19 B. An anion gap is present. The anion gap can be calculated using the formula: anion gap = $(Na^+ + K^+) - Cl^-$. Ketoacidosis will create an anion gap. With acute vomiting, H^+ and Cl^- are lost and HCO_3^- increased, resulting in metabolic alkalosis. There is no effect on the pH. This example represents a combined metabolic acidosis and alkalosis.

20 3. By convention the pulmonary artery occlusion pressure is measured at the end of expiration. In this patient who is intubated and ventilated with positive intrathoracic pressure, the wedge pressure is influenced by ventilatory cycling. Position A reflects, in part, the pressure generated by the ventilator and, therefore, does not represent wedge pressure.

21 Great debate is made about which drugs cause true anaphylaxis (IgE mediated) and which cause anaphlactoid (any nonantibody mediated hypersensitivity reaction such as direct mast cell degranulation or complement activation). Anaphylaxis and anaphlactoid are essentially immunological terms which describe the same constellation of symptoms and signs and should be considered by the clinician as the same; they should certainly be treated in the same manner.

The most common solutions and drugs known to cause anaphylaxis are:
- IV contrast media 1/2,000 (mild) – 1/40,000 (severe).
- IV dextrans or hydroxyethylated starches 1/5,000.
- IV gelatins 1/5,000.
- IV human plasma protein solution 1/10,000.
- Thiopentone 1/14,000.
- Propofol <1/1,000,000.

These incidences vary from study to study but generally are quoted in the same rank order.

Anaphylaxis requires senior assistance as this can be rapidly fatal and the airway should be secured, the patient should be ventilated with 100% oxygen. Circulatory collapse is treated with rapid infusion of crystalloid solution and a bolus of epinephrine (adrenaline) be given IV. Generally this is given in 100 μg boluses in adults, but the dose should be tailored to the response. An infusion may be required and is often recommended as a way to titrate to response, avoiding 'over treatment', specifically tachycardia and hypertension. Epinephrine is the drug of choice since it treats all of the major physiological sequelae of acute anaphylaxis. It will bronchodilate and increase vascular peripheral resistance (afterload) supporting BP. Other drugs can be used for secondary management. *They are not a substitute for epinephrine.* These include albuterol or aminophylline for bronchospasm. Hydrocortisone (500 mg) as anti-inflammatory therapy and a histamine (H_1) antagonist such as chlorpheniramine (20 mg) are frequently recommended to treat the immune response cascade. Routine blood work is rarely helpful in management, but a coagulation screen may warn of developing disseminated intravascular coagulation. Failure of clinical improvement may be noticed in two specific cases: a patient on long-term beta-adrenoreceptor blockers may be resistant to epinephrine treatment and glucagon should be considered for these patients; secondly some patients with an inherited deficiency of the C1 esterase inhibitor enzyme (hereditary angioneurotic edema) may only respond to administration of fresh frozen plasma.

22–24: Questions

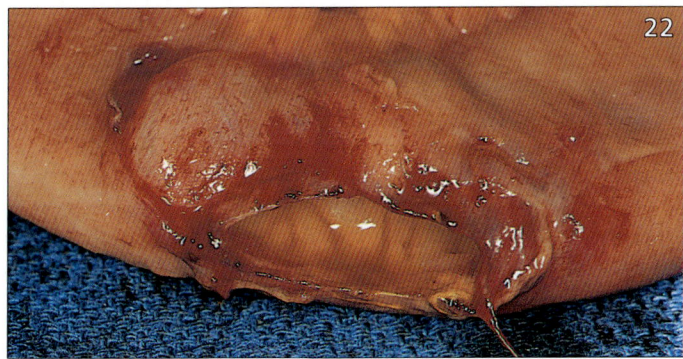

22 A 34-year-old male presented with peritonitis. His history was significant only for a 11.4 kg (25 lb) weight loss. At exploration, the source of the perforation was noted to be in the small bowel, along the antimesenteric border (**22**).
i. What is the likely etiology?
ii. Discuss his future management.

23 Persistent fetal circulation may be seen in the term or near-term infant as a result of which of the following?
A Meconium aspiration.
B Beta-hemolytic streptococcal sepsis.
C Congenital diaphragmatic hernia.
D Congenital laryngotracheal esophageal cleft.

24 A 50-year-old male (70 kg/154 lb) with short bowel syndrome has been placed on total parenteral nutrition for 1 week. The total parenteral nutrition formulation includes 400 g dextrose, 90 g protein, and 50 g lipids once weekly for a total daily calorie provision of 1,800 kcal. Physical examination of the patient is unremarkable with no signs of jaundice. The patient's vital signs are stable, and blood work reveals normal electrolytes, creatinine, and urea nitrogen. Liver function tests, obtained as part of monitoring process for total parenteral nutrition, reveal increased aspartate aminotransferase (serum glutamic-oxalacetic transaminase) and alanine aminotransferase (serum glutamic-pyruvic transaminase). The total bilirubin, direct bilirubin, gamma-glutamyltransferase, and alkaline phosphatase are normal.
i. Are the liver function tests consistent with total parenteral nutrition-induced hepatotoxicity?
ii. What are the most common hepatic complications associated with total parenteral nutrition in adults? What is the proposed mechanism leading towards this manifestation?
iii. How can this problem be managed?

22–24: Answers

22 i. This patient has a nonHodgkin (T cell) lymphoma infiltrating his small bowel and resulting in perforation. Differential diagnosis should include a complication of HIV, including cytomegalovirus infection. Treatment includes resection.
ii. When admitted for further therapy, in this case cyclophosphamide, adriamycin, vincristine, and prednisone, the patient must be carefully followed in anticipation of further spontaneous perforation.

23 A, B, and C are all classically associated with persistent fetal circulation. These were the first conditions treated with ECMO. Congenital laryngotracheal esophageal cleft is not associated with persistent fetal circulation unless there is an associated underlying cardiac or diaphragmatic defect. There have been reports of repair of congenital laryngotracheal esophageal clefts using ECMO and allowing the repair to heal without subjecting the trachea to the barotrauma from conventional ventilation postoperatively.

24 i. Total parenteral nutrition-induced liver abnormalities in adults are more frequently manifested by elevated transaminases 1–4 weeks after initiation. Elevations in bilirubin and alkaline phosphatase are less frequent, and usually occur later.
ii. In adult patients, total parenteral nutrition has been implicated to cause asymptomatic liver function tests elevation, steatosis, cholestasis, steatohepatitis, acalculous cholecystitis, and cholelithiasis. Steatosis, the more common manifestation of total parenteral nutrition-induced hepatobiliary complications, is related to the infusion of excess carbohydrate (dextrose), which stimulates insulin production. Insulin inhibits fatty acid oxidation and promotes lipogenesis, which leads to fatty deposits intrahepatically.
iii. Before deciding on a management strategy, other factors contributing to the development of hepatotoxicity, e.g. underlying diseases and medications, must be considered. In many cases, total parenteral nutrition may simply be a coincidental factor. In many instances, the continuation of total parenteral nutrition may be safely carried out as liver function tests may return to normal without clinically important sequelae. This is a viable option in this stable, asymptomatic patient. A preventive approach is to avoid overfeeding by careful nutritional needs assessment, indirect calorimetry, close monitoring, reassessment of the total parenteral nutrition formulation, and the provision of balanced macronutrients of carbohydrate, lipids, and protein. The lowering of caloric provisions from dextrose and the use of lipids may be helpful.

25–27: Questions

25 A 30-year-old female is admitted to the ICU following a motor vehicle accident. An exploratory laparotomy showed a splenic laceration, which was suture repaired, and a small pelvic hematoma. She also underwent internal fixation of her left femoral fracture. Her pelvic X-ray revealed a left superior and inferior ramus fracture. A chest X-ray revealed a left pulmonary contusion with rib fractures 4, 5, and 6. She required ventilation with 60% FiO_2, a PEEP of 10 cm/H_2O a ventilator rate of 12/min, and a tidal volume of 800 ml. She was reported to be stable during the surgical procedure. Her ventilatory pressure suddenly increases, the high pressure alarm goes off, and the patient begins desaturating. The most likely etiology is:
A Worsening pulmonary contusion.
B Pulmonary embolus.
C Fat embolism syndrome.
D Pneumothorax.
E Aspiration pneumonia.

26 What is the management of bronchospasm in a ventilated patient?

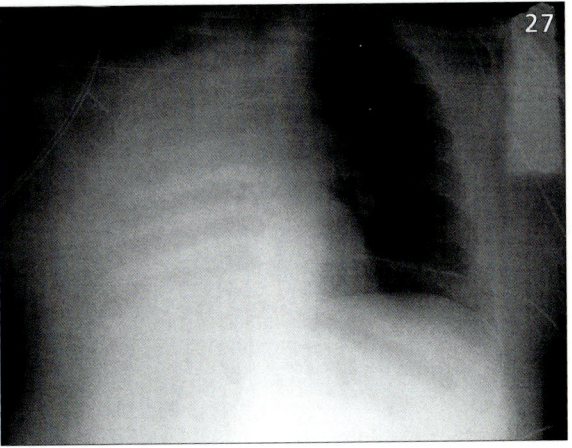

27 This 49-year-old male had an operative repair of a large ventral hernia with placement of permanent mesh. On the morning following his operation, he complained of shortness of breath. His blood gases are shown below. Examination of the chest reveals decreased breath sounds on the right.
i. What is your interpretation of these blood gases?
ii. A chest radiograph is obtained (**27**). What are your options for treatment?

PaO_2 45 mmHg (6 kPa)
PCO_2 30 mmHg (4 kPa)
pH 7.52
HCO_3^- 24 mmol/l (mEq/l)
BE +2
SaO_2 86%

25–27: Answers

25 D. The most likely etiology of sudden desaturation and increase in ventilatory pressure in a patient with blunt trauma is the occurrence of a pneumothorax. This occurs in approximately 10–20% of patients with rib fractures who are treated on positive pressure ventilation with PEEP. Some surgeons have recommended prophylactic placement of a chest tube before intubation and positive pressure ventilation. This is a life-threatening situation for an ICU patient because the pneumothorax can rapidly become a tension pneumothorax causing hemodynamic compromise. Immediate examination of the chest followed by needle aspiration and chest tube placement on the side where breath sounds are diminished is indicated. High ventilatory pressure and desaturation may be seen in the agitated patient who is biting on the oral endotracheal tube, with right main stem intubations, mucous plugging of the endotracheal tube, and bronchospasm. In the unstable patient, one should not wait for a chest X-ray to make the diagnosis of a tension pneumothorax. Worsening pulmonary contusion, fat embolism syndrome, and aspiration pneumonia, will produce desaturation and increased ventilatory pressure, but the increase in ventilatory pressure occurs over time and is not sudden. Pulmonary embolus produces desaturation but not high ventilatory pressures.

26 Simple bronchospasm should be treated by checking ET tube position and correcting if required, then by giving a beta$_2$ adenoreceptor agonist such as albuterol. This can be given directly by instilling 2.5–5 mg of nebulizer solution with some sterile saline down the ET tube and manually ventilating the lungs. This may prove difficult in the presence of significant airways obstruction and it often must be given intravenously in a dose of 3–4 mg/kg (approximately 200–300 µg for the average adult). This usually improves wheeze and oxygen saturation, but often causes significant tachycardia. Second line therapy includes aminophylline (6 mg/kg IV *slowly* over 20 minutes; average adult dose 400–600 mg), epinephrine (adrenaline) (2 mg/kg IV boluses; average adult bolus 100 µg).

If these drugs are unsuccessful, expert advise should be sought. Consideration should be given to inhaled volatile anesthetics, e.g. halothane or enflurane, nebulized local anesthetics such as lidocaine or, rarely, intravenous ketamine may be tried.

27 i. This is respiratory alkalosis with an uncorrected hypoxemia. Based on these blood gases and the clinical findings, an acute collapse of a lung segment or lobe should be suspected. These produce an acute shunt plus increased air exchange in the open lung segments.
ii. The chest radiograph shows complete collapse of the right lung with mediastinal shift. Options for treatment include intubation and ventilation, aggressive suctioning and chest physiotherapy, and bronchoscopy with or without intubation. Factors leading to this collapse should be examined, particularly the method of pain control. Placement of an epidural catheter will improve pain control and allow deep breathing and coughing. The mediastinal shift is toward the pathology which differentiates it from fluid.

28–30: Questions

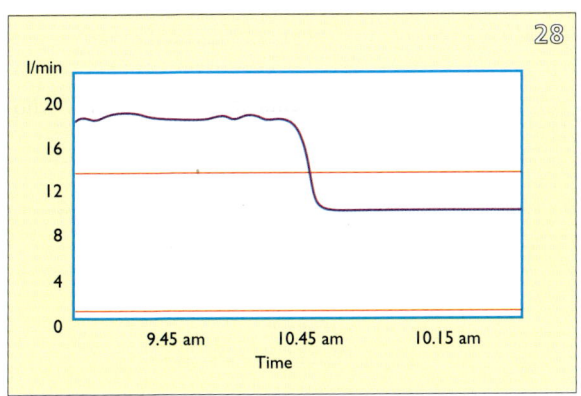

28 A septic patient receives 4 l of crystalloid solution, the response over the next 1.5 hours is seen in a continuous cardiac output trace (**28**). On the basis of this trace, what would be the next step?
A Administer 2 l of Ringer's lactate.
B Administer 2 units of blood.
C Administer steroids.
D Change antibiotics.
E Diuresis.

29 Match the following (A–I) with the correct ECG findings (1–4):
A Sinus tachycardia.
B Atrial fibrillation.
C Atrial flutter.
D Atrial flutter with variable AV conduction.
E Multifocal atrial tachycardia.
F Sinoventricular tachycardia with bundle branch block.
G Wolff–Parkinson–White syndrome.
H Atrial fibrillation and bundle branch block.
I Ventricular tachycardia.

1 Narrow QRS, regular.
2 Narrow QRS, irregular.
3 Wide QRS, regular.
4 Wide QRS, irregular.

30 A 38-year-old female presents at 37 weeks into her third pregnancy with a painless ante partum hemorrhage, having had two previous Cesarean sections. No resuscitation is required but an ultrasound scan confirms the diagnosis of major placenta praevia. A Cesarean section is performed under general anesthesia: the baby is delivered rapidly but the surgeon reports heavy bleeding and difficulty removing the placenta immediately thereafter.
i. What problems do you anticipate?
ii. How would you manage them?

28–30: Answers

28 E. This patient has gone on the down slopes of the Starling curve, leading to myocardial dysfunction. This patient has been over-resuscitated. With continuous cardiac output monitoring, this patient can be observed, assuming BP and pulse remain at an acceptable level, with the patient receiving minimal volume. Low dose dopamine may improve effective renal blood flow and allow for diuresis, moving the patient toward the top of the Starling curve. The patient was subsequently taken to surgery where an anastomotic leak was found and ileostomy performed. The hyperdynamic septic response resolved in 48 hours.

29 A and 1.
B and 2.
C and 1.
D and 2.
E and 2.
F and 3.
G and 1.
H and 4.
I and 3.

30 i. Women with major placenta praevia following previous Cesarean section can pose formidable bleeding problems, before, during, and after delivery. It is essential to be prepared for the worst case scenario, i.e. massive hemorrhage requiring Cesarean hysterectomy.

ii. Depending on the severity of the initial bleed, at least 4 units of RBCs should be cross-matched. Two large bore IV cannulae should be inserted and central venous access considered. A blood warmer should be set up: filters can be used but only if the infusion rate is still adequate. The coagulation screen should be rechecked as appropriate. If a massive transfusion is required then the FiO_2 should be increased and core temperature checked. Early liaison with the hematologist is advisable. Repeated boluses of oxytocin should be followed by an IV infusion to continue postoperatively, but IV ergometrine is a more potent oxytocic. If these fail then prostaglandins such as carboprost (Hemabate) should be given either IM or directly into the myometrium, particularly if a coagulopathy is present. Surgical measures include massage, compression, or packing of the uterus, inserting sutures in the placental bed, and early subtotal hysterectomy. Subtotal hysterectomy may be quicker and safer. Internal iliac artery ligation is commonly described but unlikely to be achieved quickly in the context of severe hemorrhage. Early hysterectomy should also be considered in the rare situation where the patient refuses blood products. Interventional radiological techniques may be helpful when surgical efforts to control bleeding have failed.

31–33: Questions

31 A 28-year-old obese male is involved in a high-speed motor vehicle crash resulting in a closed head injury, pulmonary contusion, splenic injury, acetabular fracture, and femur fracture.
i. What is the incidence of deep venous thrombosis and pulmonary embolism in this patient population?
ii. What prophylactic measures are available?
iii. What is the role of an inferior vena cava filter (31)?

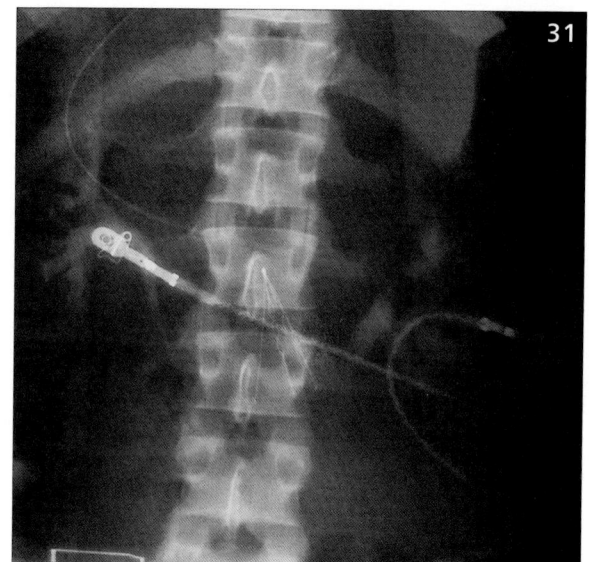

32 What hazards are associated with the use of a PEEP valve?

33 Match the description (A–C) to the formula (1–4):
A Creatinine clearance.
B Fractional excretion of sodium.
C Renal failure index.

1 $\dfrac{\text{Urine sodium}}{\text{Urine creatinine/serum creatinine}} \times 100$

2 $\dfrac{\text{Urine creatinine}}{\text{Plasma creatinine}} \times \text{volume}$

3 $\dfrac{\text{Urine sodium/serum sodium}}{\text{Urine creatinine/serum creatinine}} \times 100$

4 $\dfrac{\text{Urine osmoles}}{\text{Plasma osmoles}} \times 100$

31–33: Answers

31 i. Thromboembolic disease is a significant concern after major trauma. Risk factors include older age, blood transfusion, surgery, femur or tibia fracture, and spinal cord injuries. Without prophylaxis, impedance plethysmography can detect deep venous thrombosis in 50% of patients with major chest or abdomen injuries, 54% of head injuries, 62% of spinal injuries, 61% of pelvic fractures, 71% of tibial fractures, and 80% of femur fractures. Incriminating factors are mechanical trauma to the veins, dehydration, immobility-induced venous stasis, decrease in circulating plasmins, and an acquired antithrombin III deficiency. Fatal embolism is reported in approximately 15% of trauma patients.

ii. Pneumatic compression devices minimally augment blood return from lower extremities but exert a greater effect by increasing plasminogen release. Heparin, either in small subcutaneous doses or full systemic anticoagulation, acts by augmenting the fibrinolytic effect of antithrombin III. Studies using these modalities report lower incidence of deep venous thrombosis and pulmonary embolism but the study designs are poorly controlled. Patients with closed head injury and coma continue to have unacceptable rates of deep venous thrombosis and pulmonary embolism despite standard prophylaxis.

iii. Some authors recommend inferior vena cava filters in this population. The filter must be placed below the renal veins (**31**) because over 10% of these devices will clot causing temporary occlusion of the vena cava. Preliminary data suggest a 75% reduction in fatal pulmonary embolism for high risk patients. There is currently a need for a randomized prospective study comparing the various methods of prophylaxis.

32 Inappropriate or excessive application of PEEP is dangerous. When airway inflation pressures are already high, PEEP may cause barotrauma to the lungs or markedly decrease cardiac output by causing intrathoracic pressures that are too high. A maximum inflation pressure of no greater than 40 cmH$_2$O is recommended and ideally inflation pressures at the peak of inspiration should be much lower than this. Under certain circumstances, e.g. in hyperinflated lungs (such as in asthma) or when the potential for hyperinflation exists (such as pneumothorax), PEEP should be carefully evaluated and the effects measured before application of the PEEP valve. PEEP valves are also not as accurate as PEEP settings on a ventilator so should always be used with caution. As is common with any equipment, it may be faulty – the internal spring can stick with unwanted application of PEEP occurring. Airway pressures should always be closely monitored when using this device. Observation of the patient's chest movements to check for hyperinflation is also important.

33 A and 2.
B and 3.
C and 1.

34, 35: Questions

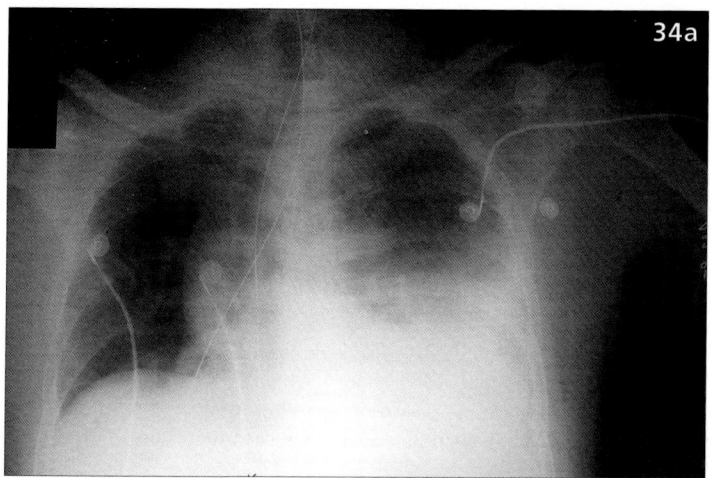

34 A 58-year-old male presented with abdominal pain and a picture of proximal-to-mid colonic obstruction. At surgery, a cecopexy is performed for a cecal bascule; however, difficulty with nasogastric tube placement is encountered. The patient later developed a fever, elevated WBC count, and a left pleural effusion.
i. The X-ray (34a) reveals the nasogastric tube placement. What would be the next appropriate step in this patient's management?
ii. What is the significance of the barium swallow, shown here (34b)?

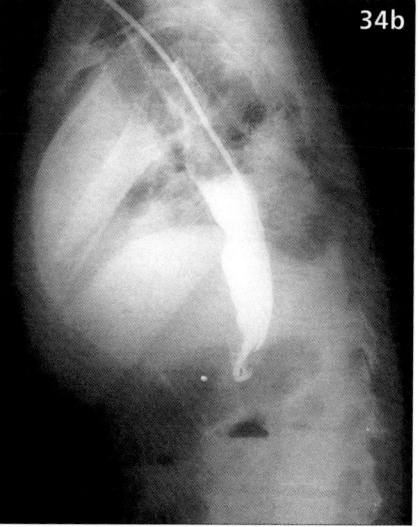

35 A 17-year-old Caucasian female presents at 34 weeks in her first pregnancy with a persistent frontal headache and generalized edema. Her BP is 180/110 mmHg (24.0/14.7 kPa) with proteinuria, 4+. A diagnosis of severe pre-eclampsia (proteinuric PIH) is made and the plan is to deliver her by Cesarean section.
i. How would you assess the mother preoperatively?
ii. What are the major risks to the mother's life?
iii. How would you prevent these complications?

34, 35: Answers

34 i. The chest X-ray revealed the initial nasogastric tube placement in the distal esophagus. Difficulty with the nasogastric tube placement should always raise the specter of gastric inlet or esophageal obstruction from stricture, tumor, volvulus, or paraesophageal hernia. Given the sudden onset of symptoms without antecedent history of gastroesophageal reflux or dysphagia, an acute process should be suspected. If the diagnosis of paraesophageal hernia is suspected, physical examination is often equivocal and other diagnostic modalities must be used. Early diagnosis of gastric volvulus or incarcerated paraesophageal hernia (as in this case) should be sought by barium swallow or esophagogastro-duodenoscopy. Systemic inflammatory signs (fever and elevated WBC count) should hasten diagnosis and definitive treatment.

ii. The barium swallow revealed a bird's beak appearance of the distal esophagus, diagnostic of distal esophageal obstruction. Abdominal distension and increased abdominal pressure caused by the bowel obstruction may have predisposed the acute incarceration of the paraesophageal hernia in a previously asymptomatic patient.

35 i. The treatment of significant pre-eclampsia in women with a mature fetus is to deliver the baby. Clinical assessment of the mother includes regular BP recordings, the severity of her edema, the presence of jaundice, epigastric tenderness, and retinal hemorrhages or hyperreflexia.

ii. Most deaths in this condition are caused by cerebrovascular consequences of the hypertension and, or, eclampsia or to pulmonary edema/ARDS. In addition, renal failure and disseminated intravascular coagulation may occur, especially in those women with HELLP syndrome (Haemolysis, Elevated Liver enzymes, Low Platelets) and there is an increased risk of thromboembolism. Remember that although the condition typically starts to improve after delivery, problems including eclampsia may arise for the first time during this period. Ideally it should be managed by a team with special experience.

iii. If the platelet count and coagulation studies are satisfactory then a regional block is preferred but many cases require general anesthesia. Severe edema may compromise the airway. Hypertension is best controlled by continuous intravenous infusion of hypotensive agents, such as labetalol. Likewise magnesium sulfate is routinely used in many centers for prophylaxis of eclampsia. Severe hypoalbuminemia may increase the patient's sensitivity to induction agents. Oliguria is due to the renal effects of the condition as well as intravascular volume depletion and is to be expected in the immediate postoperative period. IV fluids should be restricted to replacing known losses and invasive monitoring is helpful if large volumes need to be replaced. Fresh frozen plasma, cryoprecipitate, and platelet transfusions may be required but only if bleeding or severe thrombocytopenia occur. Thromboprophylaxis is appropriate: anti-embolic stockings, early mobilization, and heparin should be given.

36–38: Questions

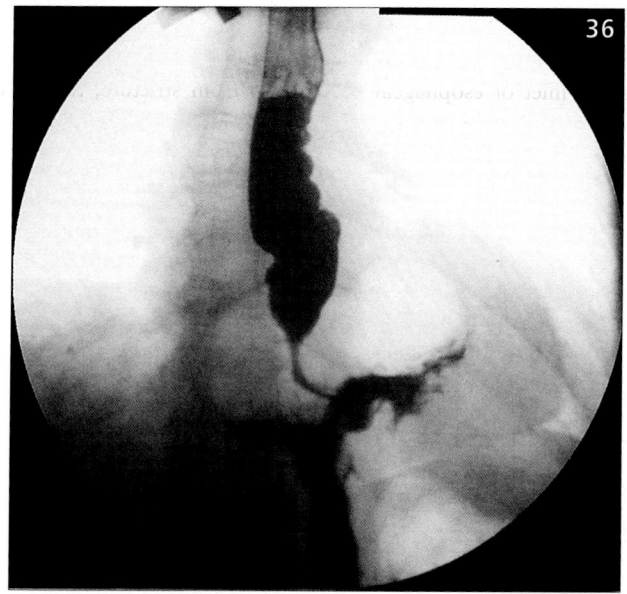

36 The patient with the shown X-ray (**36**) is best treated by:
A Gastroscopy and conservative treatment.
B Urgent surgery.
C Elective surgery in all cases.
D Elective surgery for symptomatic cases only.
E Elective surgery for cases only with reflux esophagitis.

37 A patient admitted with large lymphoma intrathoracic masses is started on chemotherapy. It is now evening and you are called because his potassium has become dangerously elevated. What can be happening and what do you do about it?

38 A 45-year-old female is booked for laparoscopic cholecystectomy for severe recurrent biliary colic. There is a family history of mesenteric infarction, venous thromboses, and pulmonary emboli. The patient has been told she is antithrombin III deficient. How should this patient be managed perioperatively?

36–38: Answers

36 D. Paraesophageal hernias with intrathoracic stomachs were in the past considered an indication for urgent surgery to avoid gastric strangulation. However, it is now recognized that gastric strangulation is rare except in symptomatic cases of obstruction. Reflux esophagitis is usually not a common symptom with this disease.

37 A syndrome of hyperkalemia, hyperphosphatemia, hyperuricemia, and hypocalcemia, called tumor lysis syndrome, occurs in rapidly proliferating tumors that undergo cell lysis. It is an oncologic emergency. Uric acid, xanthine, and calcium phosphate salts precipitate in the renal tubules leading to oliguria, acute renal failure, and lethal hyperkalemia. Although it can occur spontaneously, it is most often precipitated by cytotoxic therapy. Classically associated with the treatment of Burkitt's lymphoma, it can complicate treatment of many hematologic malignancies and some very responsive solid tumors, such as small cell lung cancer. Oliguric patients with large tumor burdens being treated with chemotherapy for the first time are most at risk. The syndrome has been reported in patients treated with steroids, tamoxifen, and interferon. Once tumor lysis syndrome occurs, calcium is replaced intravenously and hyperkalemia treated with exchange resins. A prompt nephrology consultation is desirable as severe or unresponsive abnormalities may require dialysis. The best way to manage tumor lysis syndrome is to prevent it. Patients at risk can be given allopurinol to reduce the formation of uric acid. Vigorous IV hydration, diuresis with agents such as mannitol, and urine alkalinization are maintained during the first few days of therapy to increase the solubility of uric acid while maintaining a good urine flow.

38 Antithrombin III deficiency is acquired or hereditary (heterozygous). Antithrombin III normally inactivates thrombin. Heparin binds with antithrombin III, enhancing thrombin inactivation by 750-fold, thus providing anticoagulant effect. Antithrombin III also inactivates factor Xa. Patients deficient in antithrombin III have continuous factor X activation and thrombin generation. As a result venous thrombosis occurs more frequently. This is often precipitated by surgery, infection, trauma, pregnancy, or oral contraceptives. Deep vein thrombosis, pulmonary emboli, or mesenteric vein thrombosis may be the presenting feature. Rarely arterial thrombosis occurs. Prophylaxis when asymptomatic is considered unnecessary. Prophylaxis is indicated when a risk such as surgery, trauma, or pregnancy is faced. Once a thrombotic episode has occurred, life-long anticoagulation with warfarin is indicated. Acute thrombotic episodes are treated with heparin, with monitoring of heparin levels. Heparin resistance may occur, which necessitates larger doses of heparin or administration of antithrombin III (available in concentrates or as fresh frozen plasma). In pregnancy, warfarin is contraindicated as it crosses the placenta and is teratogenic. Subcutaneous heparin in high doses during pregnancy, and antithrombin III supplements at delivery are required. Acquired antithrombin III deficiency occurs with heparin administration, disseminated intravascular coagulation, severe liver disease, and nephrotic syndrome.

39, 40: Questions

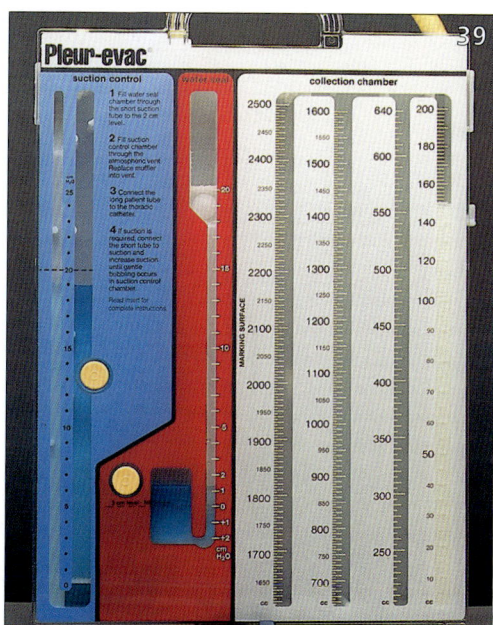

39 A 50-year-old male presents with esophageal cancer and 18 kg (40 lb) weight loss in 6 months, and poor oral intake for 3 months. He undergoes an esophago-gastrectomy. His chest tube begins to drain >100 ml/hr resulting in over 2 l of output of fluid in 24 hours (39).
i. What is your diagnosis?
ii. Why is nutrition support important to this patient's clinical recovery? (His admission serum albumin is 26 g/l [2.6 g/dl].)
iii. What three types of nutritional support could be provided for this patient?
iv. Discuss the effect water, protein, carbohydrate, and fat have on chyle production and the best source of fat for this patient.
v. How much protein would you include in this patient's nutritional regimen?
vi. What nutritional regimen would be most effective for this patient? What eventual oral diet would you recommend?

40 Standard therapy for acute status asthmaticus include all the following except:
A Inhaled beta-agonists.
B Aminophylline.
C Corticosteriods.
D Oxygen.
E Maintenance fluids.

39, 40: Answers

pH 7.57	Triglyceride 2.15 mmol/l (190 mg/dl)
Protein 28 g/l (2.8 g/dl)	Sudan stain positive
Amylase 284 u/l	Lipase 351 u/l

39 i. Based on the milky appearing intercostal catheter drainage, the diagnosis is chylous fistula. This diagnosis is confirmed by fluid analysis. Chest tube drainage was analyzed (see results above).
ii. The chyle drainage will result in large losses of fluid, electrolytes, and protein. The patient may be more predisposed to infections and poor wound healing secondary to his pre-existing poor nutritional status.
iii. 'Fat-free' (1 g/l or less) enteral nutrition formulas with high protein high carbohydrate loads, enteral nutrition with medium chain triglycerides as the sole fat source, and total parenteral nutrition with nothing by mouth.
iv. Water increases chyle flow by 20%; carbohydrate and protein have very little effect on chyle production, and dietary fats increase chyle production as much as 10-fold. Dietary fat (long chain triglycerides) is converted to chylomicron and very low density lioproteins which pass into intestinal lacteals and lymphatics then into the thoracic duct and ultimately into the venous system. An enteral product with exclusively medium chain triglycerides as the fat source is an excellent choice. Medium chain triglycerides are directly absorbed into mucosal cells without bile or micelle formation. There is no increase of chyle production. Intravenous fat emulsion is infused directly into the systemic circulation and will obviously not affect chyle production.
v. Due to increased losses from fistula drainage and the need to replete protein stores along with eventual weight gain, increased protein provision is necessary. At least 1.5 g/kg should be provided with a goal of about 2 g/kg while the fistula is healing.
vi. Total parenteral nutrition should be initiated and advanced to goal with nothing by mouth for about 2–3 weeks. Enteral nutrition with medium chain triglycerides as the fat source may begin slowly after 10–14 days and be gradually increased if no increase in fistula drainage is noted. Because of the patient's small stomach volume, the patient should receive six or more small meals per day with liquids separate from meals. An oral diet should be high in carbohydrate and fat with medium chain triglyceride supplement as the fat source.

40 B. Most studies have failed to show added benefit of aminophylline when administered with beta-agonists during the acute asthmatic episode.

41, 42: Questions

41 A 35-year-old female presents in a state of collapse in the recovery area of the operating theater 20 minutes after an elective repeat Cesarean section under general anesthesia. The procedure was apparently uncomplicated except for a transient episode of desaturation which responded to an increase in FiO_2. She is cyanosed with BP 50/20 mmHg (6.7/2.7 kPa). There is oozing from the abdominal wound.
i. What is the most likely diagnosis?
ii. How would you proceed?

42 A 65-year-old female is admitted to the cardiac ICU with unstable angina. She has cardiac catheterization through a left femoral approach which demonstrates 90% left anterior descending artery stenosis. The lesion is successfully angioplastied. Twelve hours after the procedure the nurse requests that you evaluate the patient's left groin because 'it doesn't look good' (**42a**). Auscultation reveals a bruit. A duplex ultrasound of the area is obtained (**42b**). Your diagnosis is:
A Pseudoaneurysm.
B Hematoma.
C Seroma.
D Lymph collection (lymphocele).

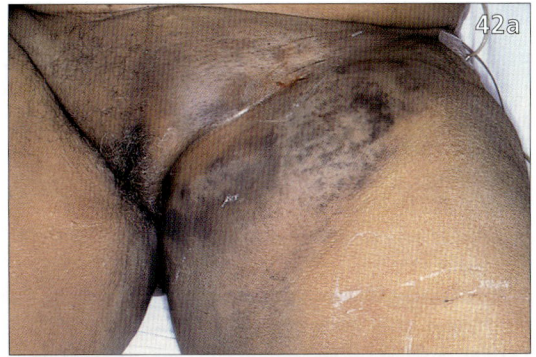

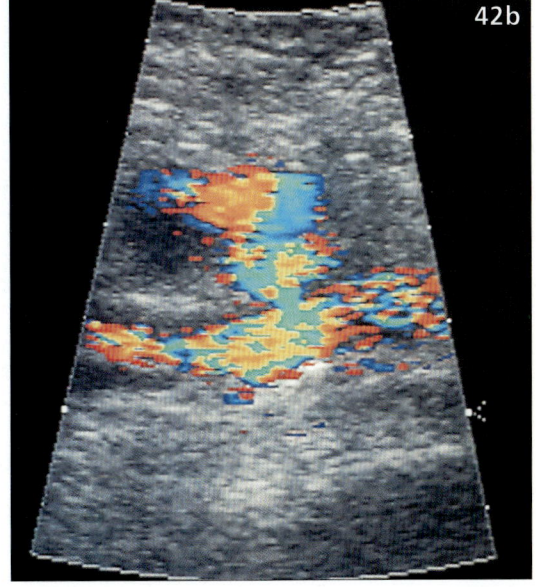

41, 42: Answers

41 i. Amniotic fluid embolism.
ii. This is a poorly understood and much feared condition. Much of what we know comes from retrospective review of fatal cases. The main features are hypoxia, cardiovascular collapse, and severe coagulation disturbance. In nonfatal cases the diagnosis is rarely confirmed.

Initial management is supplemental oxygen, possibly intubation, and ventilation. Cardiovascular support is given with fluids and inotropes as required. Disseminated intravascular coagulation may be very severe and blood products should be used to correct the coagulation disturbance. The use of heparin remains controversial and should be given on hematological advice.

42 A. The patient has a left femoral artery pseudoaneurysm resulting from the percutaneous instrumentation. Puncture site hematomas are usually not associated with bruits. The best treatment of pseudoaneurysms is prevention with careful external compression. Effective compression is difficult if the patient is obese, if the puncture site is above the inguinal ligament or below the femoral bifurcation, if there are multiple punctures of the vessel wall, and if the patient is anticoagulated or significantly hypertensive. A duplex ultrasound is the test of choice. Once the diagnosis of a pseudoaneurysm is confirmed, the ultrasound probe can be used to guide external compression of the pseudoaneurysm cavity without complete occlusion of the artery. Success in up to 80% of the cases has been reported with this approach (**42c**). Ultrasound-guided injection of thrombin has occluded pseudoaneurysms. If this fails or if the pseudoaneurysm is very tense compromising the viability of the overlying skin, then surgical repair should be strongly considered. The defect is identified and usually closed with a single stitch.

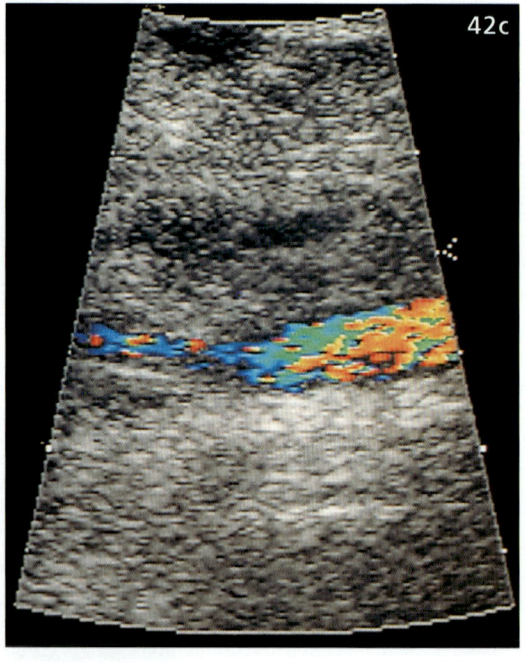

43–45: Questions

43 A concerned mother brings her 2-year-old infant to the emergency room because he is running a fever and is irritable. The physical examination is unremarkable except for an infected right ear drum with a bloody exudate. A Gram stain of the exudate is positive and shows diplococci. What is the likely causative organism?

44 Match the hemodynamics (A–D) with the clinical condition (1–5):

	A	B	C	D
BP	Decrease	Decrease	Decrease	Decrease
HR	Increase	Increase	Increase	None/decrease
CVP	None/decrease	Increase	Decrease	None/decrease
SVR	Decrease	Increase	Increase	Decrease
AVDO$_2$	Decrease	Increase	Increase	None/decrease

1 Neurogenic shock.
2 Cardiac tamponade.
3 Septic shock.
4 Cardiogenic shock.
5 Hypovolemic shock.

45 A 38-year-old patient who had a renal transplant 2 years ago is admitted to the ICU with disseminated candida septicemia and respiratory failure. Four days later the nurse notices increased abdominal distension, emesis of tube feedings, and cessation of bowel movements. A plain abdominal X-ray is taken (**45**), a rectal tube is applied, and the patient is given enemas.
i. What is your next step?
ii. What is the outcome of patients with this syndrome?

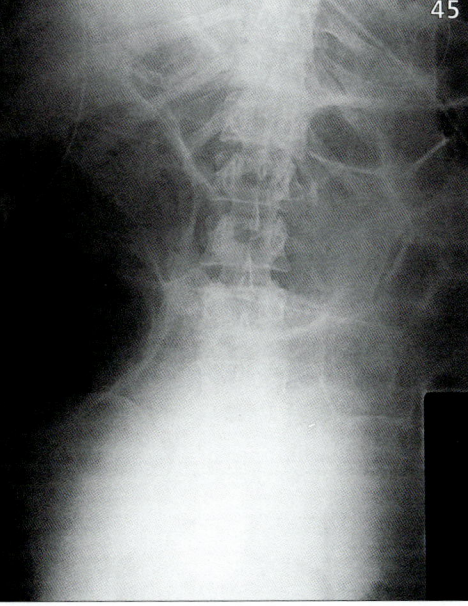

35

43–45: Answers

43 *Streptococcus pneumoniae*.

44 1 and D; 2 and B; 3 and A; 4 and B; 5 and C. There are certain recognizable hemodynamic patterns associated with shock. Hypervolemic shock is caused by a decrease in the intravascular volume relative to the vascular capacity and is generally associated with a blood volume deficit of approximately 20–25% with an even larger interstitial fluid defect. Characteristic for this picture of shock are an elevated systemic vascular resistance and a decrease in central pressures (CVP). The cardiac output is generally decreased with a hypodynamic circulation causing the increase in $AVDO_2$. A similar hemodynamic pattern is seen with both cardiac tamponade and cardiogenic shock with the exception of elevated CVPs. Cardiogenic shock is caused by an impairment in function of the pumping mechanism of the heart from acute myocardial infarction or other cardiac problems, such as cardiac tamponade. Patients with cardiogenic shock generally have a low cardiac output, increased peripheral vascular resistance, increased HR, and an increase in central filling pressures. Neurogenic shock and septic shock have a similar hemodynamic picture in that the systemic vascular resistance is low as the patient is vasodilated and pooling blood in the periphery. The patient with neurogenic shock fails to increase the HR in response to the hypotension and low systemic vascular resistance.

45 i. The patient suffers from acute colonic pseudo-obstruction (Ogilvie's syndrome), mimicking large bowel obstruction. This condition occurs after surgery of the pelvis and the hip, as well as in a variety of medical conditions including infections, CHF, stroke, respiratory failure, and metabolic abnormalities. It is characterized by a massively dilated right colon. The first step is to determine if the patient has signs of peritonitis or free air under the diaphragm, in which case a laparotomy is indicated. In cases where the cecal diameter is under 12 cm (4.7 in) a conservative approach is usually warranted, including the cessation of anticholinergic or sedative drugs, correction of metabolic abnormalities and improvement in cardiorespiratory status. The further management includes colonoscopic decompression with tube placement, percutaneous cecostomy, or laparotomy.
ii. In the absence of perforation, acute colonic pseudo-obstruction usually resolves within 3–6 days. A perforation becomes more likely if the cecal diameter exceeds 12 cm (4.7 in) and is obviously present if signs of clinical peritonitis are recognized. Risk factors for an adverse outcome are age of the patient, male sex, presence of perforation, and concomitant illnesses.

46–48: Questions

46 What are the class 2 antidysrhythmics?

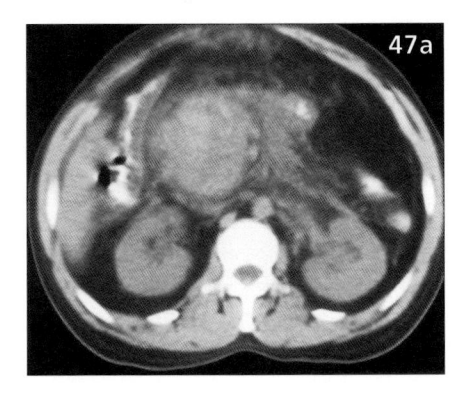

47 Interpret the CT scans of these patients with pancreatitis:
Patient A (**47a**).
Patient B (**47b**).
Patient C (**47c**).

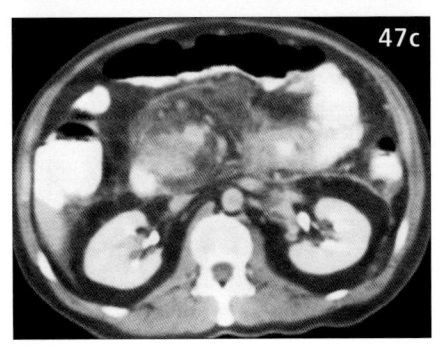

48 A 53-year-old male with a history of steroid dependent COPD, presents with sepsis secondary to a retroperitoneal abscess and back abscess. Total parenteral nutrition was initiated postoperatively secondary to ileus.
i. In addition to the provision of adequate kcal and protein, what other specific nutrients are indicated and why?
   When the above mentioned patient improved and a regular diet was 'tolerated', nutrition support and supplementation was discontinued. His wound was now in the maturation phase with active scar tissue formation. Three weeks later, however, his wound dehisced.
ii. What nutritional factor is probably involved here and why?

46–48: Answers

46 Class 2 agents include beta-blockers, which prolong A–V node conduction and depress automaticity. They can be used to treat patients with prolonged Q–T interval, with Torsades, supraventricular, and ventricular arrhythmias. Cardioselective beta-blockers have more $beta_1$ effects and may reduce the incidence of ventricular fibrillation following myocardial infarction and cardiac surgery. However, significant side effects include aggravating heart failure, heart block, and aggravating asthma or COPD.

47 Patient A: simple phlegmon.
Patient B: necrosis with air bubbles. Aspirate was sterile.
Patient C: more severe phlegmon with fluid but no necrosis.

48 i. Vitamin A is the most commonly deficient nutrient and is necessary to restore the normal inflammatory response. For wound healing, a provision of 20,000–25,000 units/day for 10 days is recommended (except in the presence of renal failure) for anyone on steroids or with pre-existing nutrition deficiencies. Zinc stores are frequently depleted with steroid use and there are excessive urinary losses in the presence of stress. It is necessary for nucleic acid synthesis, cell replication, protein synthesis, and collagen formation. A 220 mg capsule or 10–15 mg IV for 10–14 days is appropriate. Vitamin C is critical for the hydroxylation of proline, necessary for collagen synthesis and chemotaxis of neutrophils and macrophages. It also protects iron and copper from oxidation. Supplementation of 1–2 g daily initiated within the first 24 hours decreases the degradation of intracellular collagen and increases collagen production.
ii. Given that the nutrition support and supplementation was discontinued, it is possible that he did not have adequate vitamin C, which can become depleted rapidly in the body without adequate intake. The maturation process of wound healing involves continuous collagen reorganization (i.e. collagenase activity continues to break down collagen and collagen production should also continue). In the presence of a vitamin C deficiency, collagen production decreases contributing to tissue degradation. Vitamin C supplementation of 1–2 g daily should continue through the maturation process of wound healing.

49–51: Questions

49. How can the NADH/NAD ratio be used to determine the degree of tissue hypoxia?

50 A 42-year-old male with third-degree burns covering much of his chest and arms is admitted to the hospital. Two days later his fever reaches 40°C (104°F). His blood culture grows colonies of Gram-negative rods that are oxidase-positive, produce a blue-green pigment, and smell like 'grapes'. What is the likely causative organism?

51 The chest X-ray presented (51) is that of a 24-year-old female following a motor vehicle accident. The patient is hypotensive with a BP of 90/60 mmHg (12.0/8.0 kPa) and a pulse of 130/min. The accident was described as a high energy impact/head on collision and the patient was entrapped by her lower extremities for approximately 20 minutes There are obvious significant orthopedic injuries including a mid-shaft femur fracture and bilateral open tibial fractures. The patient fails to stabilize after 2 l of crystalloid infusion, the application of MAST trousers and 2 units of PRBCs. A diagnostic peritoneal lavage is clear/colorless. Subsequent evaluation reveals a significant third-thoracic process.
i. What is your differential diagnosis?
ii. What confirmatory diagnostic approach(es) might be considered?
iii. Discuss operative options.

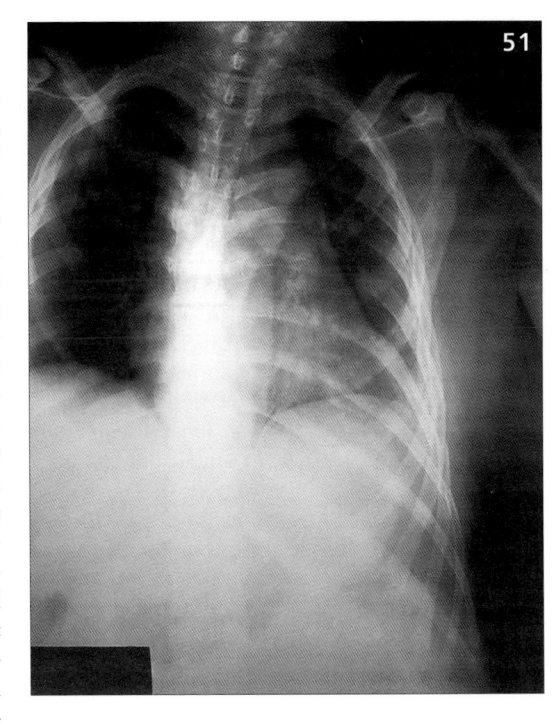

49–51: Answers

49 NAD is a coenzyme that can be reduced to $NADH_2$. Under aerobic conditions $NADH_2$ can be oxidized. Under anaerobic conditions NAD is reduced to $NADH/NADH_2$. The ratio (or redox state) of tissue can be reflected by the following formula:

$$\frac{lactate}{pyruvate} = \frac{(NADH)(H)}{(NAD)}$$

Thus increases in $NADH/NADH_2$ over NAD imply increasing hypoxia. This can be easily measured in experimental models by spectrometry, biopsy, or assay.

50 *Pseudomonas aeruginosa*.

51 i. The patient has sustained a blunt rupture of the right atrium with resultant cardiac tamponade. The X-ray demonstrates normal thoracic landmarks. The pericardial silhouette is unremarkable. The pericardium does not accommodate acutely and significant hemodynamic compromise can occur in patients with a radiographically normal cardiac silhouette. The diagnosis of cardiac injury with tamponade should be considered in the patient who has suffered significant blunt force trauma and fails to respond to standard resuscitation measures. Concomitant intra-abdominal hemorrhage, orthopedic, and neurologic injuries must be rapidly assessed and addressed. Clinical signs associated with cardiac tamponade include muffled heart tones, jugular venous distension, and hypotension (Beck's triad).
ii. The placement of a CVP monitoring line may distinguish this entity from other traumatic etiologies. In the setting of cardiac tamponade the CVP is elevated in contradistinction to traumatic hypovolemic hemorrhagic shock. Pericardiocentesis may provide transient improvement but should not delay preparation and transport to the operating room.
iii. Rapid drainage of the pericardium via a subxiphoid pericardial window improves hemodynamic stability if tamponade is severe. This approach also definitively establishes the diagnosis of tamponade and may be accomplished rapidly under local anesthesia. The decompression afforded by subxiphoid window improves tolerance of general anesthesia for formal cardiac repair. If severe hypotension, intractable ventricular arrhythmia, or cardiac arrest occurs at any point during the resuscitation, a left anterior thoracotomy is immediately performed and pericardial decompression quickly accomplished. Median sternotomy provides excellent exposure for control and definitive repair of the majority of cardiac injuries. Repair of intracardiac shunts and valvular injuries can almost always be deferred for elective repair.

52–54: Questions

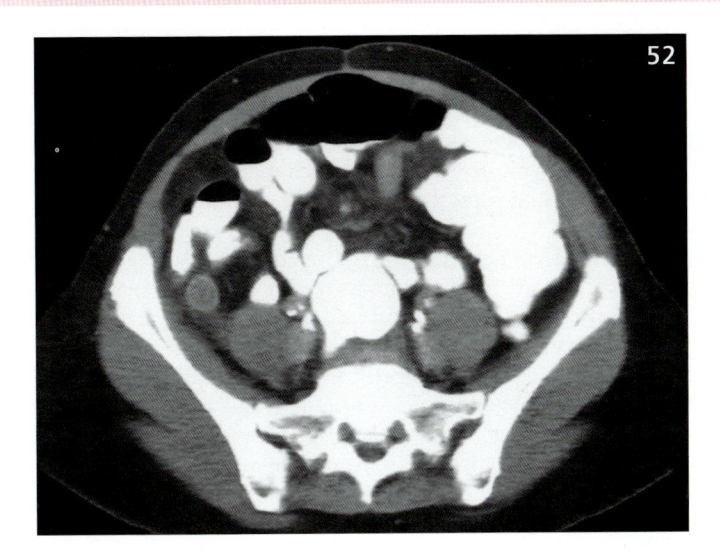

52 This patient presented with abdominal pain, mainly in the right lower quadrant, with mild diarrhea and only mild nausea. He has a history of HIV and *Pneumocystis carnii* pneumonia. His CT is shown (52). Discuss the management of this case.

53 A 62-year-old black male is admitted to the hospital with severe pancreatitis. His past medical history is significant for alcoholism, diabetes mellitus, pancreatitis and upper gastrointestinal bleeding. Drug and food allergies include anaphylaxis to sulfa and egg products. The patient is 165 cm (5 ft 5 in) tall and weighs 45.6 kg (100 lb 8 oz). Laboratory data are shown.

| WBC 20 x 10⁹/l (20,000/mm³) |
| Lipase 450 u/l |
| Hemoglobin 100 g/l (10 g/dl) |
| Triglycerides 6 g/l (600 mg/dl) |
| Amylase 650 u/l |
| Blood glucose 20 g/l (360 mg/dl) |
| Albumin 25 g/l (2.5 g/dl) |

i. What options for nutritional intervention are appropriate in this patient?
ii. Discuss the use of IV fat emulsions in pancreatitis.
iii. List several complications associated with the use of IV fat emulsions.

54 A 75-year-old male has oliguria following resection of an infrarenal aortic aneurysm. Given the data shown, what conclusions can be drawn regarding intrinsic renal function?

| Urine Na⁺ 65 mmol/l (mEq/l) |
| Plasma Na⁺ 145 mmol/l (mEq/l) |
| Urine creatine 2,475 μmol/l (28 mg/dl) |
| Plasma creatine 211 μmol/l (2.4 mg/dl) |

52–54: Answers

52 This patient has appendicitis. In HIV patients, who have abdominal pain but in conjunction with chronic diarrhea, no nausea, and evidence of AIDS, a CT scan is useful as up to 75% of the time the problem is not a surgical one. Common etiologies include viral colitis and the morbidity of a negative laparotomy can be high. However, if there is a typical presentation such as pain that migrates to the right lower quadrant, nausea and focal tenderness, a CT scan is not absolutely needed.

53 i. Either total parenteral nutrition and, or, jejunal tube feeding with an 'elemental' type product is appropriate, until symptoms resolve and the patient can be gradually advanced to an oral diabetic diet. Enteral feeding has the advantages of reduced cost, ease of delivery, prevention of bacterial translocation, and fewer complications.
ii. IV fat emulsions are not contraindicated in patients with pancreatitis. If the blood specimen is noted as lipemic and, or, has a serum value of >18 mmol/l (>500 mg/dl) after infusion of 500 ml over 24 hours, patients should receive this product only to prevent essential fatty acid deficiency. This particular patient has an allergy to eggs resulting in anaphylaxis. IV fat emulsions should not be used in patients with known egg allergies, since the emulsion is composed of egg phospholipids derived from egg products.
iii. Immediate (acute) <1% incidence include: dyspnea, cyanosis hyperlipemia, hypercoagulability, nausea, vomiting, headache, flushing, temperature elevation, sleepiness, chest and back pain, and dizziness. Long term (chronic): hepatomegaly, jaundice due to central lobular cholestasis, splenomegaly, thrombocytopenia, leukopenia, transient elevation in liver function tests, fat overload syndrome, focal seizures, fever, leukocytosis, splenomegaly, and deposition of brown pigmentation in the reticuloendothelial system.

54 The calculated fractional excretion of sodium (FENa) is >3%, as calculated by the formula:

$$FENa\% = \frac{\text{urine } Na^+/\text{plasma } Na^+}{\text{urine creatine}/\text{plasma creatine}} \times 100$$

Values <1% imply prerenal azotemia, while values >3% imply abnormal renal function, including early acute tubular necrosis. However, the true volume status relative to cardiac function cannot be assessed without further information.

55–57: Questions

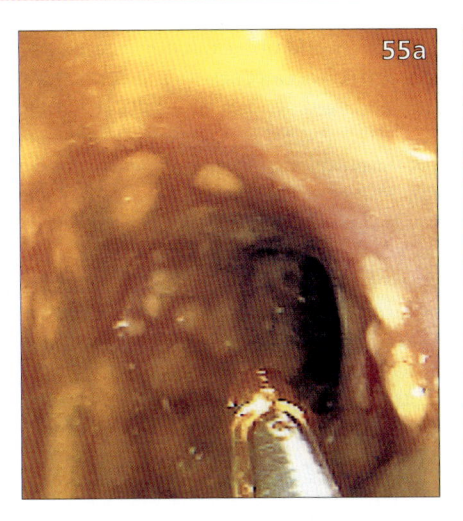

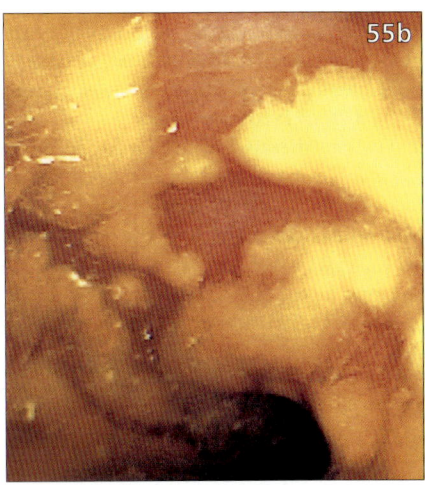

55 A 66-year-old female is treated with IV antibiotics for pneumonia. She complains of watery nonbloody stools and crampy abdominal pain 6 days later. Stool studies are ordered and the gastroenterologist performs a flexible sigmoidoscopy without preparation and finds the abnormality shown (55a, b).
i. What is your diagnosis?
ii. How would you treat the patient?
iii. The patient was discharged from the hospital and readmitted to the hospital 5 days later with increased abdominal pain, fever but improved diarrhea. What is the diagnosis?

56 A 72-year-old male who has suffered a cardiac arrest 6 hours ago is intubated. He has a radial arterial line and a Swan–Ganz catheter in place. Discuss two different methods of determining cardiac output in this patient.

57 The characteristics of congenital benign bronchoesophageal fistulas are:
A Best treated by endoscopic techniques.
B Best treated by thoracotomy and division of the fistula.
C Usually present with symptoms in adulthood.
D Due to esophageal inflammation.
E Usually having a connection between the bronchus and the cervical esophagus and are best treated by a cervical approach.

55–57: Answers

55 i. The picture shows pseudomembranous colitis, a condition caused by the Gram-positive bacterium *Clostridium difficile*. This is a primarily nosocomial infection and a frequent cause of antibiotic-associated diarrhea. The diagnosis is usually made by using a stool cytotoxin assay.

ii. The first therapy should be discontinuation of the antibiotic therapy. Patients with *C. difficile* colitis are generally treated with an antibiotic capable of eradicating the bacterium from the stool. Both vancomycin and metronidazole can be used. Metronidazole has become the first choice in many institutions due to a cost advantage.

iii. Relapses after successful therapy are common. Reintroducing antibiotic therapy is one risk factor. Given this scenario a toxic megacolon as a consequence of the colitis needs to be considered. A plain radiograph should be obtained, which in this case demonstrated a dilated colon and thickening of the bowel wall. In cases of a moderately severe relapse a second course of antibiotics is warranted, however, the presence of an acute abdomen or failure to improve after medical therapy calls for a surgical approach.

56 The reverse Fick method and thermodilution method are two ways of determining cardiac output. The reverse Fick equation is used if whole body oxygen consumption can be measured by analysis of inspired oxygen and expired oxygen by indirect calorimetry. Oxygen consumption is then divided by the difference of the arterial and mixed venous oxygen content:

$$\text{cardiac output (l/min)} = VO_2/AVDO_2$$

This method can only be used in steady state and when no type of right-to-left or left-to-right shunt exists. The thermodilution method determines cardiac output when a Swan–Ganz catheter is in place. A thermistor is at the tip of the Swan–Ganz catheter which is inserted in the pulmonary artery. Cardiac output is determined when a known amount of saline (10 ml) at a known temperature (4°C/39.2°F) is injected in the right atrium along with venous blood returning to the heart. The venous blood and cold saline is mixed in the right ventricle where it then flows through the pulmonary artery and thermistor. The Stewart–Hamilton formula is then used to calculate cardiac output:

$$\text{cardiac output} = (V[T_b-T_1]K_1K_2)/ \Delta T_b(t)dt$$

where V = injected volume, T_b = blood temperature, T_1 = injectate temperature, $\Delta T_b(t)dt$ = change in blood temperature as a function of time, and K_1 and K_2 are constants.

57 C. Congenital bronchoesophageal fistulas are due to a fistula between the bronchus and the middle one-third of the esophagus. Almost all are present in adulthood and should be treated by thoracotomy, division, and interposition of a flap to prevent reformation of the fistula.

58–60: Questions

58 A 50-year-old male is seen with right arm swelling and mental status changes of 24 hours in duration. He had a fall 5–7 days ago. On examination, his temperature is 38.7°C (101.7°F), he is confused, his HR is 120/min, and his RR 30/min. Examination reveals a swollen forearm

| Hemoglobin 157 g/l (15.7 g/dl) |
| WBC 24.9 × 10⁹/l (24,900/mm³) |
| Urea 20.2 mmol/l (BUN 121.4 mg/dl) |
| Creatinine 283 µmol/l (3.2 mg/dl) |
| Lactate 6.9 mmol/l (mEq/l) |

with pulses at the wrist. Laboratory data are shown. Does this patient fit the diagnosis of sepsis syndrome, systemic inflammatory response syndrome, or septic shock?

59 Match each of the following scenarios (A–D) with the electrolytes measurements for cases 1–4:
A Volume contraction secondary to vomiting.
B Volume contraction secondary to diarrhea.
C Volume contraction secondary to diuretics.
D Volume contraction secondary to osmotic diuresis.

Case	Serum Na^+ [1]	K^+ [1]	HCO_3^- [1]	Cl^- [1]	Urine Na^+ [1]	Cl^- [1]	Osmolality [2]
1	140	3.0	33	97	40	10	600
2	149	3.0	22	117	70	100	320
3	133	2.9	35	88	60	110	500
4	140	3.3	18	112	10	10	800

[1] mmol/l, mEq/l   [2] mmol/kg, mOsm/kg

60 A 75-year-old male is admitted to the ICU in septic shock. After initial resuscitation, the patient is taken for a CT scan (60). What are the causes for this abnormality?

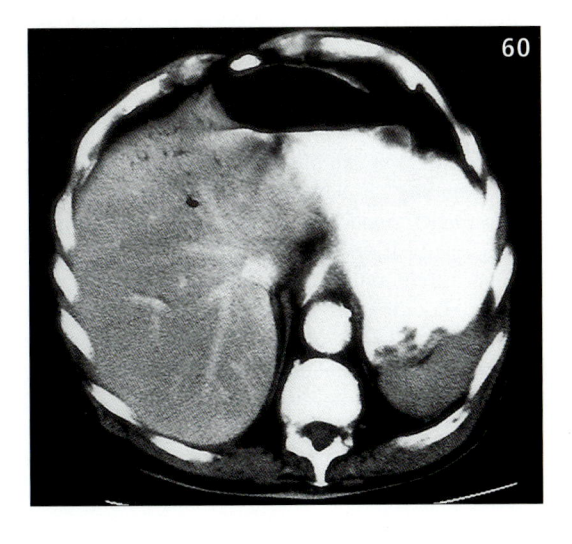

58–60: Answers

58 All three. At this point in the patient's evaluation, you can definitely say he is showing evidence of systemic inflammatory response syndrome. He must meet at least two of the following criteria for systemic inflammatory response syndrome:
- Temperature >38°C (>100.4°F) or 36°C (96.8°F).
- HR >90/min.
- RR >20/min or PCO_2 <32 mmHg (<4.3 kPa).
- WBC >12 × 10^9/l (>12,000/mm^3) or <4 × 10^9/l (<4,000/mm^3) or >10% bands and he meets all four of them.

The definition of sepsis is: systemic inflammatory response syndrome with a documented infection. As this patient's forearm appears to be infected, he fits this criteria also. Septic shock is defined as sepsis associated with organ dysfunction, hypoperfusion, or hypotension. Although the patient's BP and urine output are not given in this example, he is confused – an indication of organ dysfunction, and his lactate level is 6.9 mmol/l (mEq/l), indicating tissue hypoperfusion. He is septic and in shock.

59 A and 1; B and 4; C and 3; D and 2. *Acute vomiting*: volume loss occurs with acute vomiting. Loss of H^+, a metabolic alkalosis, occurs with a low serum K^+. Although volume contraction occurs the urine Na^+ may be increased because excess HCO_3^- acts as a nonabsorbable anion and prevents maximal Na^+ conservation. The low urine Na^+ is caused by the acid loss with vomiting and Na^+ re-absorption from urine. *Diarrhea*: diarrhea fluid loss leads to a volume contraction or dehydration. The kidney conserves Na^+, Cl^-, and water. The urine Na^+ <20, urine Cl^- low, and urine osmolality is high. The diarrhea fluid contains high levels of K^+ and HCO_3^-. This base loss stimulates renal acid secretion and increase ammonia in the urine. *Diuretics*: diuretics promote water, Na^+, K^+, and Cl^- loss in the urine. Metabolic alkalosis occurs. Thiazide diuretics may produce an electrolyte profile similar to the syndrome of inappropriate secretion of antidiuretic hormone. *Osmotic diuresis*: osmotically active particles produce large water loss in the urine in excess of Na^+ (polyuria). This polyuria leads to volume contraction and elevated serum Na^+. K^+ wasting occurs. The urine Cl^- is greater than the urine Na^+ and the serum osmolality equals urine osmolality.

60 This patient has pneumobilia. A CT scan is the most sensitive study for pneumobilia, although it can also be found using ultrasound, nuclear study, or plain film. The classic finding on plain films of the abdomen is the 'Saber sign' which is produced by air in the left hepatic duct and can be seen in about 50% of patients. Rarely, hepatic artery calcifications can be mistaken for pneumobilia on ultrasound examination.

The differential diagnosis for pneumobilia includes: spontaneous internal biliary fistula, incompetent sphincter of Oddi, emphysematous cholecystitis, and biliary enteric bypass. This patient as described most likely has a fistula or emphysematous cholecystitis and warrants an operation.

61–63: Questions

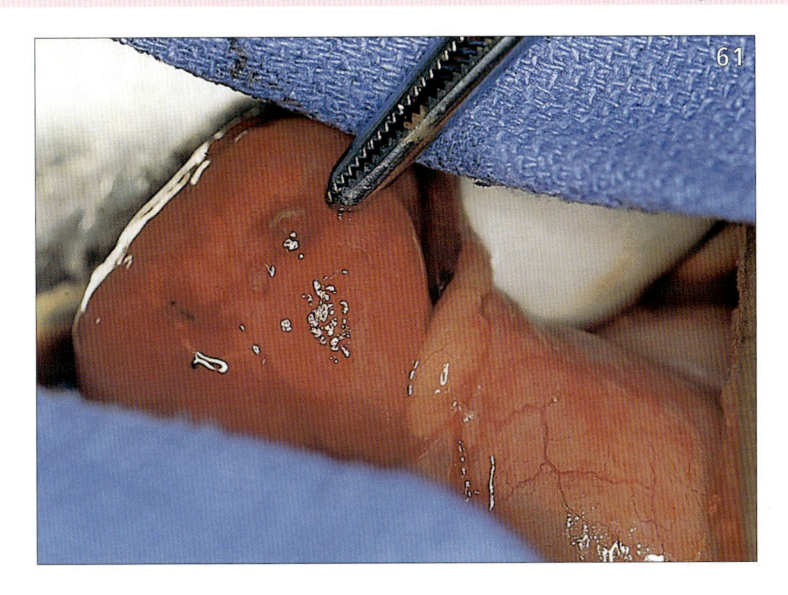

61 A 41-year-old male presented with massive hematemesis. Endoscopy suggested a pin point mucosal lesion in the cardia (**61**). Wedge resection of this area was carried out and the gross and microscopic appearance confirmed the diagnosis of a 'Dieulafoy' lesion. Briefly discuss this lesion.

62 A well-nourished, 26-year-old white male has received a severe trauma to the head. Pentobarbital infusion has been initiated.
i. Describe two different methods to determine resting energy expenditure.
ii. Which method is the most accurate?
iii. If the Harris Benedict equation is used to calculate resting energy expenditure, what would be the approximate dose reduction factor as a percentage of total calories for this patient?
iv. Discuss the mechanism(s) of action for barbiturate reduction of resting energy expenditure.
v. What are the general protein requirements based upon g/kg ideal bodyweight in this patient population assuming normal renal and hepatic function?

63 A 19-year-old male army recruit awakens one morning during basic training with a stiff neck and a fever of a 40.2°C (104.4°F). You suspect meningitis and perform a spinal tap. A Gram stain of the spinal fluid reveals Gram-negative diplococci and many neutrophils. What is the causative organism?

61–63: Answers

61 Dieulafoy 'ulcers' are vascular malformations, that occur within 6 cm (2.4 in) of the gastroesophageal junction, usually along the lesser curve, and are associated with massive recurrent bleeding. The abnormally large vessel runs just under the gastric mucosa and the endoscopic appearance varies from normal to a visible protruding vessel. Medical management is usually not successful or appropriate. Surgery usually entails a wedge resection.

62 i. Resting energy expenditure (REE) can be calculated using the Harris Benedict equation and multiplying the basal energy expenditure (BEE) by an injury factor (IF).

Harris Benedict equation:

male:	BEE = 5(H) + 13.75(W) + 66.43 − 6.78(A) = Kcals/day
female:	BEE = 1.85(H) + 9.65(W) + 655.1 − 4.68(A) = Kcals/day

where H = height in cm; W = weight in kg; A = age in years.

Resting energy expenditure:

$$REE = BEE \times IF$$

A second method is indirect calorimetry, obtained using a metabolic cart which measures VO_2 consumption and carbon dioxide (VCO_2) production to determine energy requirements based upon the relationship of gas exchange and the metabolism of nutrients.

ii. Indirect calorimetry is the most accurate tool available to assess energy requirements and the body's physiologic response to the provision of fat, carbohydrate, and protein.

iii. Barbiturate therapy decreases energy expenditure to 14% below predicted.

iv. The CNS effects of barbiturates result in a decrease in energy expenditure by suppressing neurons that control systemic metabolism, suppression of neuronal activity associated with decerebrate rigidity in muscle tone, hypothalamic alterations in temperature regulation, glucose metabolism, and sympathetic mechanisms.

v. Increased nitrogen excretion continues for several weeks after head injury, regardless of aggressive calorie and protein provision. During this hypercatabolic phase, head-injured patients need 1.75–2.0 g/kg of protein/day based upon ideal body weight.

63 *Neisseria meningitidis.*

64, 65: Questions

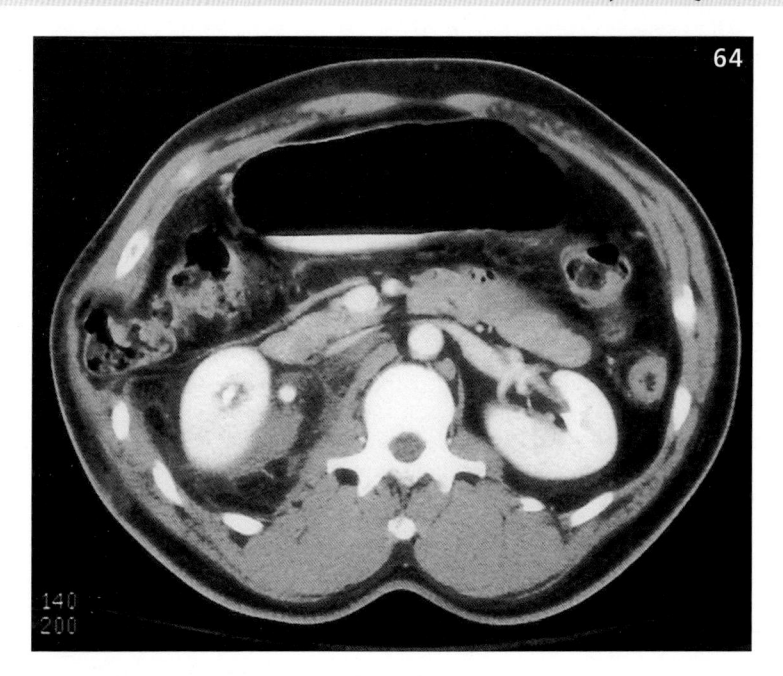

64 A 23-year-old male was hit by a motor vehicle. He is hemodynamically stable but complains of a right-sided chest and abdominal pain. His initial chest radiograph was interpreted as normal. An image from his abdominal CT scan is shown (64).
i. What abdominal injury is suggested by this image?
ii. What are the current methods for diagnosing and treating this condition?

65 With regard to congenital diaphragmatic herniae, which of the following is/are true?
A *In utero* surgical correction of the defect is the ideal treatment for the majority of congenital diaphragmatic herniae.
B Surgical repair is best done when the infant has been successfully weaned from ECMO/ECLS.
C Laparotomy or thoracotomy and urgent surgical repair of the diaphragm should be undertaken regardless of ventilatory status.
D ECMO/ECLS should be necessary in less that 50% of congenital diaphragmatic herniae.
E ECMO/ECLS via either arterial venous or veno–venous cannulation should be instituted when 'conventional ventilation' fails to maintain a postductal PaO_2 >100 torr.

64, 65: Answers

64 i. The CT scan reveals bowel, most likely colon, in the soft tissues of the right thoracoabdominal region, indicating that the diaphragm has been ruptured. The diaphragm is injured during severe anterior–posterior compression. Associated injuries exist in 75–90% of blunt trauma cases. The most common injuries are pelvic fracture, head injury, and rib fractures as well as liver and spleen injuries.
ii. The diagnosis requires a high index of suspicion. Indirect evidence is seen on the chest radiograph only 50% of the time. Herniation of the stomach with a coiled nasogastric tube in the left chest is the most obvious sign. An irregular, elevated, or indistinct diaphragmatic border may also be present. Diagnostic peritoneal lavage is notorious for missing this injury. CT scans have a low sensitivity for this injury. MRI is felt to have a high sensitivity but the scarcity, slow speed, and cost of these studies renders them impractical. Endoscopy, either thoracoscopy or laparoscopy, are the most definitive tests. Laparoscopy is best suited for hemodynamically stable victims of blunt trauma with suspicious chest radiographs but no other indication for laparotomy. All detected diaphragmatic ruptures should be repaired. The natural history is for the lacerations to increase in size over time because of the continual tension during respirations. Repair should be undertaken with a nonabsorbable suture. The repair is most often carried out via an abdominal incision as this allows for repair of associated injuries. In this particular case, there is also an intercostal hernia with disruption of the fascia between the eighth and ninth ribs.

65 B and D. Although *in utero* surgery is undertaken for congenital diaphragmatic herniae in a very few select pediatric and neonatal centers, one must still consider this a relatively experimental treatment, and at this time it would not be considered the standard. The majority of congenital diaphragmatic herniae which are symptomatic in the first 24 hours of life should be successfully managed with means other than ECMO. Conventional ventilation with nitric oxide and other ventilatory modes such as high frequency oscillatory ventilation may be all that is required. Where these fail and the child's oxygenation and ventilation are deteriorating, then ECMO should be instituted. Standard protocols are used to decide which infants are appropriately managed this way and it is a decision made jointly with the neonatalogist, cardiologist, surgeon, and radiologist. Veno–venous or arterial venous may be used; an $AaDO_2$ value >600 mmHg (>80 kPa) or an oxygenation index >25 are accurate predictors of mortality and hence the need for ECMO. Because of problems with anticoagulation and hemodynamic instability, procedures are best done following successful weaning from ECMO. Morbidity and mortality are adversely affected by urgent surgical repair of the diaphragm in an unstable child with compromised ventilation and oxygenation.

66, 67: Questions

66 A 49-year-old male presents to the ICU in septic shock with complaints of increasing rectal pain. Two days before his admission, he underwent incision and drainage of a perirectal abscess in an outpatient setting and was placed on antibiotic therapy. The perineum is shown (**66a**).
i. What is this condition called and what therapy would you prescribe?
ii. After initial surgical debridement and stabilization of the patient in the ICU, what else must be done?

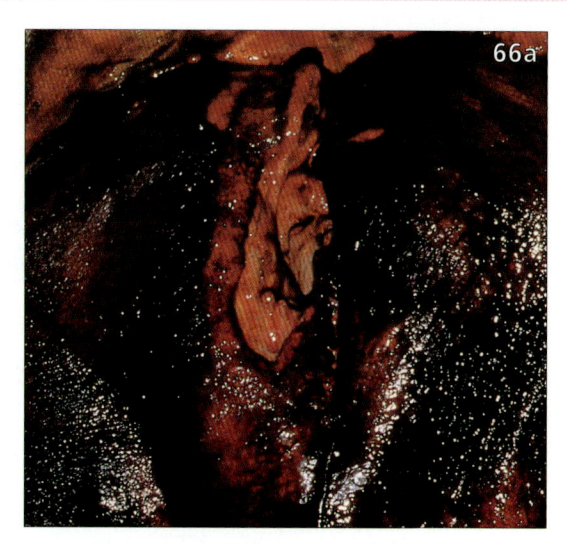

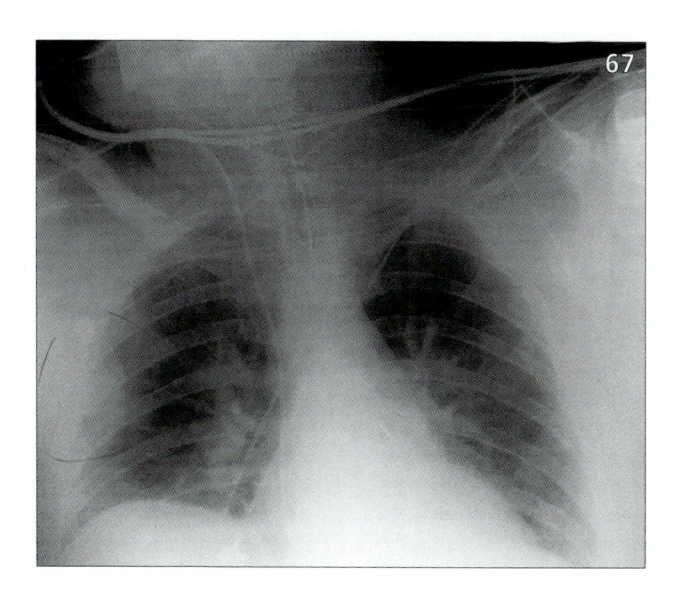

67 During elective femur surgery, a 48-year-old male develops increasing oxygen requirements and is unable to be extubated postoperatively. His initial chest X-ray is normal but he continues to have evidence of pulmonary hypertension and increased alveolar–arterial gradient. The day following surgery, this chest X-ray is obtained (**67**). What is the abnormality identified?

66, 67: Answers

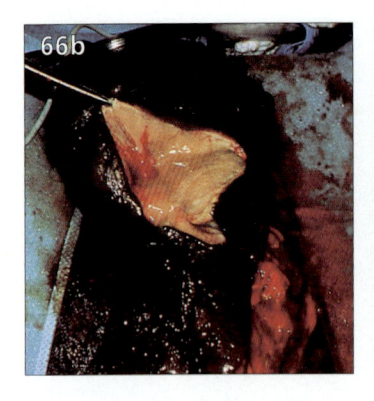

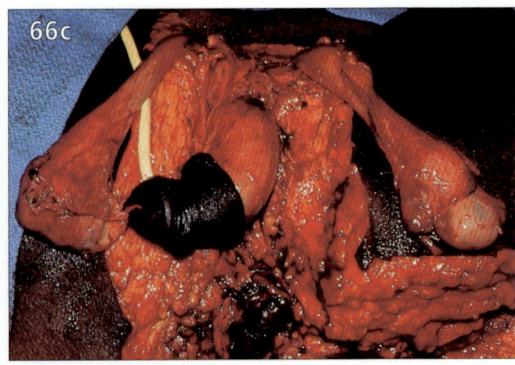

66 i. This is perineal gangrene which was first described by Fournier in 1883. Fournier's gangrene is defined as a fulminant rapidly spreading infection of the scrotum that also involves the perineum, penis, and abdominal wall (**66b**). This necrotizing infection is a synergistic polymicrobial infection, usually related to pathology in the colorectal or genitourinary system. The mortality rate is approximately 22%. The treatment involves resuscitation, broad-spectrum antibiotics directed by tissue cultures, and aggressive surgical debridement. Initially debriding of the gangrenous tissue to healthy tissue (**66c**). Multiple debridements may be required along with accompanying procedures including colostomies and suprapubic cystostomies. After control of the sepsis, skin grafting over the area may be required.

ii. A careful search for the etiology of the patient's problem must be performed. Colorectal disease (33% of cases) includes anorectal or ischiorectal abscesses, perianal fistulas, prolapsed hemorrhoids, anal fissures, perforated diverticulitis, and perforated rectal carcinoma. Genitourinary tract disease (21% of cases) includes prostatic infections, urethral obstruction, epididymitis, phimosis, periurethral abscess, traumatic urethral catheterization, extension of bladder carcinoma, urethral rupture, thrombosis of the dorsal vein of the penis, and hydrocele. Soft-tissue trauma from bites, injections, or previous surgery have also been reported as possible etiologies. These underlying conditions may influence the outcome of the patient with perineal gangrene and must be diagnosed and treated during the same hospitalization. The diagnosis may require CT scanning, cystogram, or exploratory laparotomy. The cause of this man's perineal gangrene was a perirectal fistula.

67 Although hidden by overlying bony structures, there is a wedge defect in the periphery of the lung field. An angiogram confirmed the presence of a pulmonary embolism.

68, 69: Questions

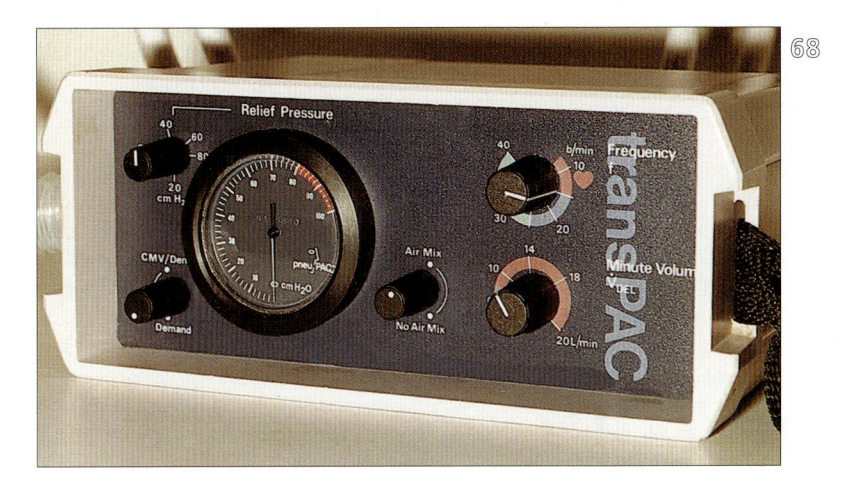

68 i. What is this piece of apparatus?
ii. How would you set it to work in the trauma bay?
iii. What can go wrong with it?

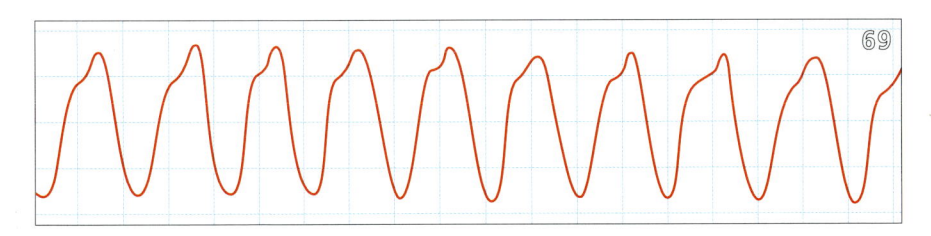

69 A 45-year-old female with a history of depression, anxiety disorder, and schizophrenia presents to the emergency department unresponsive with seizures. The patient was found in bed with multiple empty pill bottles scattered in the bedroom. Vitals are temperature 37.2°C (99°F), pulse 110/min, BP 82/50 mmHg (10.9/6.7 kPa), and RR 12/min. The ECG is shown (**69**).
i. The patient's symptoms are most consistent with an overdose of:
A Sertraline hydrocholoride.
B Amitriptyline.
C Buspirone.
D Haloperidol.
ii. What are the ECG manifestations of tricyclic overdose?

68, 69: Answers

68 i. This is a simple ventilator for use under temporary circumstances in areas such as the trauma bay or in a transport vehicle. It is a simple minute volume divider.
ii. All that is set is: whether the patient is to breathe 50% air/oxygen mix or 100% oxygen; the required minute volume; the rate or frequency of breaths.
iii. There are few things that can actually go wrong with the ventilator *per se*; however, some basic knowledge is required of ventilation: (1) The average tidal volume for adults is approximately 10 ml/kg. For the 'average' person a tidal volume of 700 ml is reasonable. The average number of breaths is 10–15, therefore tidal volume × number of breaths = minute volume. Thus reasonable initial settings for this ventilator under emergency conditions is 7–10 l/min with the number of breaths being 10–15/min. (2) Patient airway pressures and chest wall movements *must* be checked when the ventilator is first attached to the patient. High airway pressures are particularly dangerous (i.e. over 40 cmH_2O) and may cause a pneumothorax. High airway pressures can also result from bronchospasm, a kinked, blocked or misplaced (particularly in the right main bronchus or at the carina) endotracheal tube. The patient must be closely observed to see whether ventilation and the chest wall movements seem appropriate. The lungs should be auscultated, to check for abnormal breath sounds. A pulse oximeter should be attached and saturations of <90% should cause concern. End-tidal CO_2 is also extremely helpful in determining adequacy of ventilation, the normal range being 4.6–6.0 kPa (35–45 mmHg).

69 i. B. Tricyclic medications are used to treat many conditions including depression, obsessive-compulsive disorders, chronic pain syndromes, peripheral neuropathies, and nocturnal enuresis. There is a narrow range between therapeutic and toxic effects. TCAs exert several distinct pharmacological actions. Inhibition of amine uptake results in tachycardia, hyperreflexia, seizures, and rigidity. Antagonism of muscarinic receptors can cause delirium, coma, and anticholinergic symptoms. Na^+ and K^+ channel blockages result in cardiac conduction abnormalities and arrhythmias. Inhibition of alpha-receptors causes hypotension. GABA receptor antagonism can result in seizures. TCAs are lipophilic and have a large volume of distribution. Less than 2% of ingested TCA is found in the bloodstream, therefore, serum levels are not an accurate predictor of toxicity. The normal half-life of TCAs is 24 hours but can be as long as 72 hours in an overdose situation. Clinical manifestations include CNS depression, anticholinergic symptoms, respiratory depression, hypotension, seizures, and cardiac conduction abnormalities.
ii. Possible cardiac arrhythmias include, sinoventricular tachycardia, ventricular tachycardia, premature ventricular contractions, and conduction blocks. ECG manifestations include tachycardia, right axis deviation, and prolongation of the PR, QRS, and QT intervals. Treatment involves standard supportive care for coma, seizures, and hypotension. Ventricular arrhythmias can be treated with lidocaine, bretylium and cardioversion. Class IA and IC antiarrhythmics, beta blockers, calcium channel blockers, and phenytoin are contraindicated in the treatment of TCA induced arrhythmias. Alkalinization therapy with sodium bicarbonate is indicated for QRS complex widening >100 ms, hypotension refractory to fluid challenges and ventricular arrhythmias.

70–72: Questions

70 A 63-year-old male, ventilated in the ICU following a laparotomy for a perforated duodenal ulcer, develops hypotension and a reduced urinary output. He requires insertion of a pulmonary artery flotation catheter to guide fluid management and possibly treat a low cardiac index. Describe what is seen on the invasive pressure monitor as the pulmonary artery catheter is inserted to wedge in the pulmonary capillary. Such a description is best given in diagrammatic form.

71 A 33-year-old black female with sickle-cell disease has had flu-like symptoms for the past 3 days. On the afternoon of her admission she was feverish with a shaking chill and fainted. When she arrived at the emergency room she was febrile, hypotensive, and had a tachycardia. A blood culture was performed and empiric antibiotic treatment with ampicillin, gentamicin, chloramphenicol, and nafcillin sodium was initiated. The laboratory results showed alpha-hemolytic colonies of Gram-positive, lancet-shaped diplococci that were inhibited by optochin. What is the causative organism?

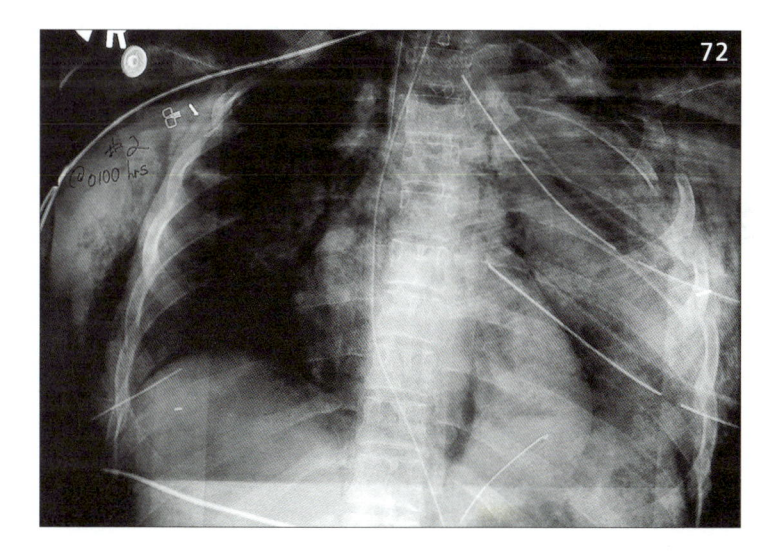

72 The tracheobronchial injury from blunt trauma shown in the X-ray (**72**) is likely to be:
A Most commonly transverse and in the trachea.
B Most commonly transverse and in the left main bronchus.
C Most commonly transverse and in the right bronchus.
D Most commonly longitudinal and in the thoracic trachea.
E Most commonly longitudinal and in the left main bronchus.

70–72: Answers

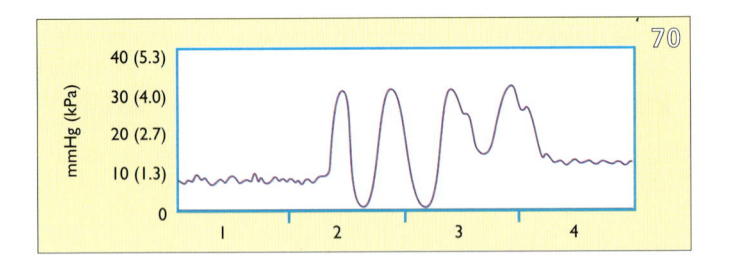

70 See tracings 1–4 (**70**). (1) *CVP/right arterial tracing*: normally 5.0–7.0 mmHg (0.7–0.9 kPa). This is usually found after 15–20 cm (6–8 in) of catheter insertion. The balloon on the pulmonary artery catheter should now be inflated. The catheter *must* only be advanced with the balloon up. There are three components to the waveform found in the central venous system: a, c, and v. The 'a' wave represents atrial contraction; the 'v' wave the closure of the mitral valve; and the 'c' wave represents ventricular contraction. These are rarely seen in practice. (2) *Right ventricular tracing*: this usually displays a pressure of 20–40/0–5 mmHg (2.7–5.3/0–0.7 kPa) and is usually found as the catheter is inserted to 25–35 cm (10–14 in). (3) *Pulmonary artery tracing*: this is characterized by the presence of a dichrotic notch on the downslope of the arterial trace. The development of a significant diastolic pressure occurs with a reading typically of 20–40/10–15 mmHg (2.7–5.3/1.3–2.0 kPa). It is entered at around 35–50 cm (14–20 in). (4) *Wedge tracing/pulmonary artery occlusion pressure*: this resembles reappearance of the central venous waveform and indicates that the catheter is 'wedged' in the pulmonary artery. The pressure at this level reflects the filling pressures of the left side of the heart. The catheter should not be advanced any further as it may go on to rupture the pulmonary artery. The wedge pressure should be less than the pulmonary artery diastolic pressure typically around 12–15 mmHg (1.6–2.0 kPa) in an optimally fluid resuscitated patient with no vasoconstrictor or PEEP therapy. Once the balloon is deflated a pulmonary artery trace should reappear. If this does not happen the catheter should be withdrawn by about a centimeter and the balloon reinflated. Pressure fluctuations will occur with respiration. Pulmonary artery occlusion pressures should be read at the end of the expiratory phase of both spontaneously breathing and positive pressure respiration, bearing in mind that the appearance of the tracings will be different depending on whether the patient is ventilated or not.

71 *Streptococcus pneumoniae*.

72 C. Bronchogenic tears caused by blunt trauma are most commonly transverse and occur in the right main bronchus. Review has shown that these tears are usually transverse 74% of the time versus longitudinal 17% of the time. Of the transverse tears, 4% are in the cervical trachea, 12% are in the thoracic trachea, 25% in the right main bronchus, 17% in the left main bronchus, and 16% are in a lobar bronchus.

73–75: Questions

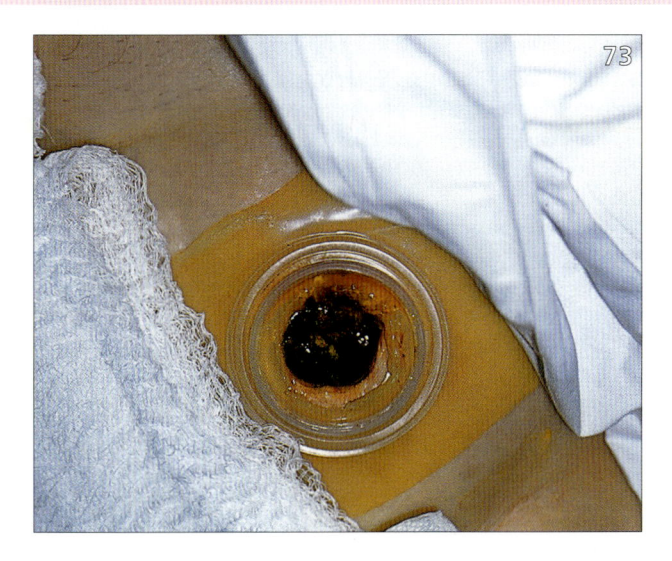

73 This ileostomy (73) was created for a patient who required a right colectomy for a perforated cecum. How would you evaluate this problem?

74 A 23-year-female is brought to the emergency room after being caught in a fire in her apartment. Her vital signs are: HR 135/min, BP 75/palpable mmHg (10.0 kPa), and RR 36/min. She is unconscious and sustained third degree burns to her face and chest. She is wearing black nail polish on her fingers. Resuscitation is begun and the patient is orally intubated and mechanically ventilated with 100% oxygen. A pulse oximeter is applied to her finger and reads 78%.
Reasons to account for the low oxygen saturation by pulse oximetery include:
A Systemic hypotension.
B Carbon monoxide poisoning.
C Smoke inhalation injury.
D Black fingernail polish.

75 A victim in a roll-over accident in mid-winter was trapped in his motor vehicle. He complained of lower back pain and being short of breath. There is no immediate hazard such as fire and the patient is conscious. Discuss the initial approach and possible sequela.

73–75: Answers

73 The bluish discoloration of the ileostomy indicates a compromised blood supply. A test tube can be inserted into the depth of the stoma to determine the color of the underlying mucosa above the fascia. If the mucosa is pink, the stoma will survive and urgent reoperation is not required. However, if the entire mucosa is blue, early reoperation is required to revise the ileostomy. Technical problems during the formation of the ileostomy commonly lead to this picture and include a twisting of the mesentery, excessive tension on the mesenteric blood supply to the ileostomy, and removal of too much mesentery at the terminal end of the ileostomy. Under-resuscitation of a septic patient can lead to low cardiac output and this picture. The use of vasopressors to maintain a blood pressure will constrict the arterial supply to this ileostomy. Unrecognized, the superior mesenteric artery thrombosis or embolization can also cause bluish discoloration of the ileostomy. These factors leading to low cardiac output or low blood flow to the ileostomy must be evaluated and addressed.

74 All of the above. Pulse oximeters measure arterial oxygen saturation, which is physiologically related to oxygen tension by the oxyhemoglobin dissociation curve. Low perfusion states such as systemic hypotension from hypovolemia result in reduced perfusion to the extremities and may lead to false oximeter readings. However, the threshold of decreased perfusion that leads to misleading recordings has not been clearly defined. As a result, the oximeter reading may still represent a true level of arterial desaturation despite the degree of hypotension. Other causes of arterial desaturation, such as smoke inhalation injury, must therefore be sought. Fingernail polish with absorbencies at the same wavelengths used by the oximeter sensor (660 and 940 nm) may produce falsely low readings. This includes blue, green, and black nail polish. The problem can be avoided by placing the oximeter probe on the finger side-to-side rather than front-to-back. Carboxyhemoglobin has an absorption spectrum similar to oxyhemoglobin and, therefore, may be misinterpreted by the oximeter as oxyhemoglobin. As a result, oximeters overestimate the true oxygen saturation in the presence of carboxyhemoglobin. In all cases where there is uncertainty as to the accuracy of the pulse oximeter readings, blood gas analysis of PaO_2, and, if necessary, arterial oxygen saturation by co-oximetry should be performed.

75 Emergency services personnel often have to extract patients from nearly impossible circumstances. In this case the vehicle was buried in snow and unstable. The snow had to be dug away and the vehicle supported and elevated with blocks and air bags. The victim had to be extracted carefully due to suspected lumbar sacral spine injuries, and during the prolonged extrication was supported with oxygen and blankets. Because of the length of time this took he developed hypothermia and required intensive external warming en route to hospital.

76–78: Questions

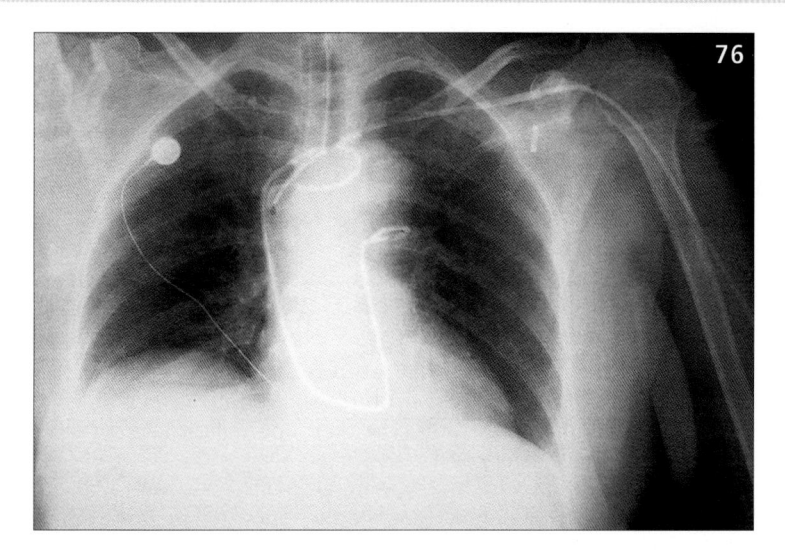

76 This chest radiograph (**76**) represents the position of a pulmonary artery catheter. Placement of this catheter was reported to be difficult. What is the problem? The pulmonary capillary wedge pressure was achieved at 75 cm (30 in) of insertion.

77 A 3-year-old female is brought to the emergency department by her grandmother. She reports that the child was found sitting on the bedroom floor with an open bottle of baby aspirin at her side. The bottle is now empty, but the grandmother states it was a new bottle which was full yesterday. Salicylate levels have been ordered. What is the earliest time that the Done nomogram can be used to determine degree of toxicity: 2, 4, 6, or 8 hours?

78 Effective therapies for the treatment of status epilepticus includes all the following except:
A Succinylcholine.
B Phenytoin.
C Phenobarbital.
D Benzodiazepines.
E Pentobarbital.

76–78: Answers

Access site	Right atrium	Distances cm (in) Right ventricle	Pulmonary artery
Right internal jugular vein	20–25 (8–10)	25–30 (10–12)	30–35 (12–14)
Left internal jugular vein	20–25 (8–10)	30–35 (12–14)	35–40 (14–16)
Right subclavian vein	20–25 (8–10)	25–30 (10–12)	30–35 (12–14)
Left subclavian vein	20–25 (8–10)	30–35 (12–14)	35–40 (14–16)
Right femoral vein	40–45 (16–18)	45–50 (18–20)	50–55 (20–22)
Left femoral vein	45–50 (18–20)	50–55 (20–22)	55–60 (22–24)

76 The pulmonary artery catheter has been inserted to an extreme length and has coiled within the heart. This is a technical problem with insertion and should have been recognized at the time of insertion. The chart above illustrates the distances to the pulmonary artery from various access sites.

77 Six hours. Aspirin is found in hundreds of prescription and nonprescription medications. Because of its widespread availability, both accidental and intentional overdoses are common. ASA is metabolized in the liver. In overdose situations metabolism reaches zero order elimination and renal excretion becomes an important route of elimination. ASA stimulates the respiratory centers of the CNS resulting in a respiratory alkalosis but also inhibits the production of blood buffers causing a metabolic acidosis. Signs and symptoms of ASA toxicity include nausea and vomiting, hematemesis, abdominal pain, hyperventilation, diaphoresis, tinnitus, CNS changes (confusion, lethargy, seizures, coma), coagulation disorders, hyperthermia, dehydration, pulmonary edema, and cardiac arrhythmias (ventricular tachycardias, premature ventricular contractions, and ventricular fibrillations). Serum levels <150 mg/kg are considered nontoxic. Levels between 150–300 mg/kg are considered moderately toxic. Serum levels >300 mg/kg are graded as severe toxicity. The Done nomogram can be used to predict toxicity. It can only be used after a single acute ingestion in which no salicylates have been taken within the last 24 hours. Levels drawn before 6 hours cannot be used to predict toxicity. The nomogram cannot be used in acute overdose situations in which ASA was taken over several hours. It also cannot be used in chronic ASA poisoning or after the ingestion of enteric coated ASA. Treatment involves supportive care, hydration, and alkalinization of blood and urine. Blood pH should be kept >7.4. Hemodialysis is indicated in cases of severe cardiac or neurologic toxicity, renal failure, pulmonary ARDS, inability to successfully alkalinize urine, or deterioration despite aggressive supportive care.

78 A. Neuromuscular paralysis is contraindicated in seizure control.

79–81: Questions

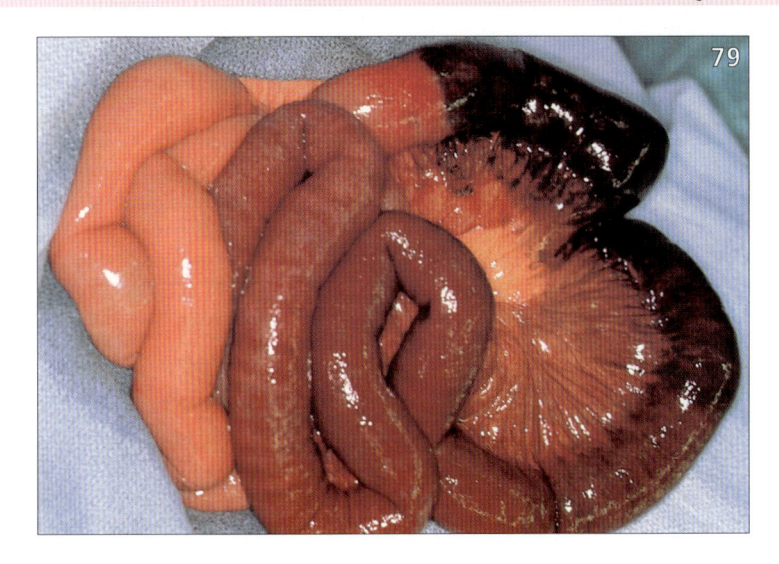

79 What are the clinical and laboratory findings that are associated with this finding on laparotomy (79)?

80 The patient you are seeing in clinic concluded six cycles of cyclophosphamide, adriamycin, vincristine, and prednisone chemotherapy for a lymphoma about 2 months ago achieving a complete remission. Laboratory studies today reveal a hemoglobin of 60 g/l (6 g/dl). Work-up for anemia is not necessary since the patient's hemoglobin can be explained by the recent chemotherapy. True or false?

81 A 63-year-old male presented with increasing liquid stools (>1,000 ml/day) and general malaise. He was discharged 1 week ago. During the previous admission, he had a distal ileal resection with end-to-end ileocolon anastomosis. He was discharged on a regular diet.
i. What steps would you take to confirm that this is an osmotic vs. secretory diarrhea?
ii. Why is osmotic diarrhea probable?
iii. How would you treat this patient?

79–81: Answers

79 Intestinal ischemia, if due to bowel obstruction, is usually associated with obstructive symptoms and a radiographic pattern that demonstrates dilated small bowel. Nonobstructive intestinal ischemia, usually associated with mesenteric emboli or thrombosis, is often more subtle. History of atrial fibrillation, the use of digoxin, and vascular disease should be sought. Clinically, the predominant early features are of severe, poorly localized, pain out of proportion to physical findings. With time there may be progression to abdominal distension, heme positive stools, and finally shock with peritonitis. Abdominal X-rays may reveal bowel wall edema, thumb printing, pneumatosis, or air in the biliary tree. Blood tests are nonspecific but can include elevated serum lactate, hemoconcentration, elevated amylase, but most predominately a severe leukocytosis.

80 False. Most chemotherapy regimens produce only mild changes in hemoglobin from which patients should recover when the treatment has concluded. While extended duration of chemotherapy with agents such as cisplatin can result in a chronic anemia for which some have advocated use of erythropoietin, a hemoglobin level below values associated with anemia of chronic illness should prompt a search for other etiologies.

81 i. Make the patient 'nil by mouth'. Osmotic diarrhea usually responds with a decreased stool volume within 24 hours. Secretory diarrhea will continue despite 'nil by mouth' status. Check the stool osmolality and osmotic gap. Stool osmolality for secretory diarrhea is usually about the same as serum osmolality (280 mmol/kg [mOsm/l]). Osmolality with osmotic diarrhea will be less.

Stool osmotic gap = measured stool osmolality − 2 × (stool Na^+ + stool K^+).

The gap with osmotic diarrhea is usually 160 mmol/kg (mOsm/kg) or more. Secretory diarrhea usually has a small to negative osmotic gap. Check the stool culture for bacteria, *Clostridium difficile*, WBC, and fecal fat. Fecal fat results may be dilutionally false. (A true fecal fat test involves stool collection for 3 days with concurrent intake of 80–100 g fat/day.)
ii. There are two primary reasons. First, the distal ileum is the primary absorptive site for bile salts bound to fat. When these are not reabsorbed, they can cause an osmotic influx of water into the colon upon presentation there causing steatorrhea. Secondly, this patient's removal of the ileocecal valve, otherwise, known as the 'intestinal brake', causes rapid entry of small bowel content into the colon.
iii. Once stool cultures are confirmed negative, antidiarrheal medication can be initiated. The appropriate diet with this type of fat malabsorption is low fat with supplemental medium chain triglyceride oil. A multiple vitamin with minerals preparation should also be initiated.

82–84: Questions

82 You are treating a hypertensive patient with indistinct epigastric abdominal pain and have taken an X-ray (**82**). He describes a tearing sensation which goes through to his back and his nurse mentions that his BP is 200/120 mmHg (26.7/16.0 kPa). What diagnosis do you suspect and how would you treat this?

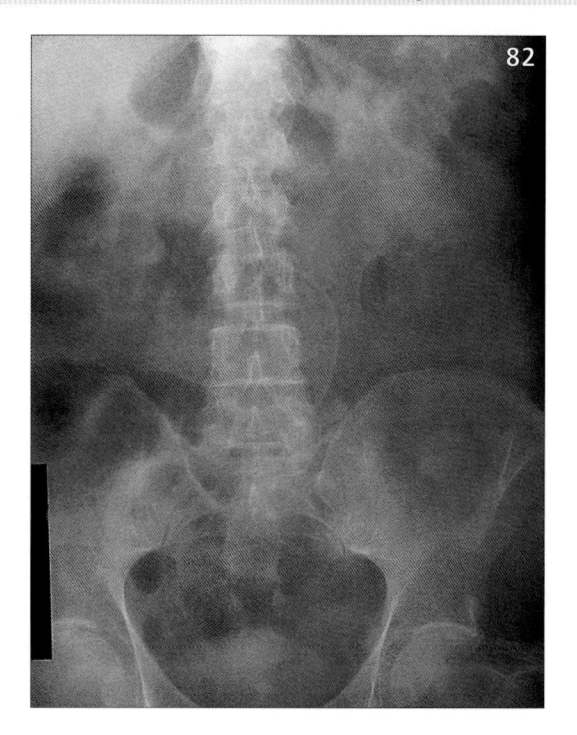

83 A 7-year-old male is taken to the ICU postoperatively after having undergone a laparotomy for a perforated appendix. He has a history of an uncorrected tetralogy of Fallot. One hour after admission to the ICU, he begins to awaken from anesthesia. His oxygen saturation, which had been running 87% falls precipitously to 58%. The ventilator is set in assist control mode with a rate of 15/min, tidal volume of 450 ml, 100% oxygen and PEEP at 0. Appropriate interventions to improve this patient's oxygenation include which of the following:
A Intravenous administration of morphine.
B Inhalation of nitric oxide at 20 p.p.m.
C Intravenous administration of propranolol and neosynephrine (phenylephrine).
D Infusion of dobutamine at 5 µg/kg/min.

84 Each of the following topical antimicrobial agents is associated with well known undesirable side effects. Enumerate for each: silver sulfadiazine, mafenide acetate, and silver nitrate.

82–84: Answers

82 The plain X-rays of this patient demonstrate a calcified aorta which looks aneurysmal. His pain could be caused by a slow rupture of his aortic aneurysm because of a hypertensive crisis. Appropriate pharmacologic management of this patient is similar to that of acute aortic dissection. The two forces associated with rupture are the mean arterial pressure and the pulsatile flow (dp/dt). Priorities are for short acting and reversible agents, in case the patient does rupture. Nitroprusside is an excellent first line agent for reduction of BP, but it can increase dp/dt when used alone. Other options are ganglionic blockade, direct vasodilation, and calcium channel antagonism. Specifically for dp/dt, beta-adrenergic blocking agents are very good negative inotropes with esmolol being an easily titrated short-acting option.

83 A and C. Tetralogy of Fallot includes four anatomic features: a ventricular septal defect, right ventricular outflow tract obstruction, an overriding aorta, and right ventricular hypertrophy. The greatest concern is the presence of a hypertrophic pulmonary infundibulum, which, if spasm occurs, will lead to a hypercyanotic crisis. Spasm may result from increased myocardial contractility, which, in turn, may result from agitation, hypovolemia or tachycardia. Treatment of a hypercyanotic spell should include 100% oxygen and placement of the patient in a knee-chest position may prove beneficial. The patient should receive morphine for sedation and IV fluid should be given to ensure an adequate circulating blood volume. The systemic vascular resistance can be elevated with a phenylephrine infusion and contractility can be reduced with beta-blockade. Nitric oxide is a selective pulmonary vasodilator. It has no proven role in the management of hypercyantoic spells.

84 Silver sulfadiazine is associated with a nonspecific leukopenia, with WBC counts often decreasing to the $3 \times 10^9/l$ (3,000/mm^3) range. Mafenide acetate is associated with a carbonic anhydrase effect and resulting metabolic acidosis. Topical silver nitrate is associated with sodium and chloride disturbances, the most severe being a hypernatremia. This agent is not often used now because of the two cream preparations above. However, on occasion, it is useful when silver sulfadiazine or mafenide acetate is contraindicated because of allergic responses.

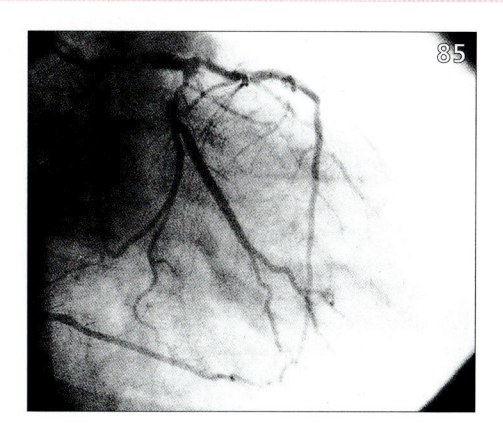

85–87: Questions

85 A 68-year-old male suffers a non-Q myocardial infarction following a laparotomy for perforated duodenal ulcer. His recovery is complicated by mild CHF but not by angina. Echocardiography reveals his ejection fraction to be 25% with generalized hypokinesia, anteroapical myocardial thinning, and mild mitral regurgitation. Coronary angiography shows (85): 95% stenosis of the LAD with 80% narrowing of the first diagonal, 90% narrowing of the proximal circumflex, and occlusion of his RCA which reconstitutes well distally. Thallium scanning shows large areas of reversible ischemia in the lateral and inferior distributions. Discuss the indications, timing, and results of coronary artery bypass grafting in this patient.

86 Match the complication (A–D) to the diuretic (1–4).
A Produces rebound intracranial hypertension.
B Produces metabolic acidosis.
C Produces a decrease in potassium, magnesium. Produces decreased serum levels of potassium, magnesium, and calcium.
D Increases serum lipid levels.

1 Acetazolamide.
2 Furosemide (frusemide).
3 Mannitol.
4 Thiazide.

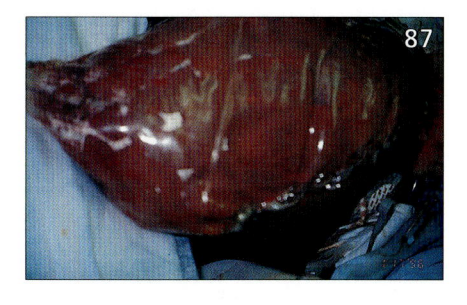

87 A 28-year-old male suffered a gun shot wound to the chest. In the operating room he had a repair of a cardiac injury, repair of a diaphragmatic injury, hepatorrhaphy, and repair of transverse colon and small bowel lacerations. During the procedure he received 8 units of packed RBCs and over 10 l of crystalloid. Currently, he is tachycardic, hypotensive, and oliguric. No response to fluid boluses is noted. A postoperative chest X-ray shows only surgical changes. His abdomen is distended with no bowel sounds. He is returned to the operating room for a procedure (87). Discuss the etiology of the patient's hypotension and oliguria.

85–87: Answers

85 This patient with three-vessel coronary artery disease, severely reduced ventricular dysfunction, and evidence of hibernating or stunned myocardium, will undoubtedly benefit from a coronary artery bypass graft. Optimal timing of surgery is less certain, although non-Q infarction with demonstrable ischemia is an unstable situation with a 5% hospital mortality. Death is more likely when angina is present and still more likely when angina occurs in the presence of ECG changes. Thus a coronary artery bypass graft is recommended during the same hospital admission. Results of surgery in this situation depend upon comorbidities as well as the patient's age, but most would quote an operative mortality of approximately 3–5%. Survival at 5 years should be more than 90% (compared to 60% for medical therapy). The effect of a coronary artery bypass graft on ventricular function in this situation is unpredictable. It is likely that this patient would experience substantial improvement in ventricular function and perhaps complete resolution of his mitral regurgitation.

86 A and 3. Mannitol is an osmotic diuretic used for the treatment of increased intracranial pressure. Mannitol may result in a paradoxical increase in intracranial pressure several hours after the dose. The mechanism of this rebound pressure is unknown, but may relate to delayed entry of mannitol into the cell.

B and 1. Acetazolamide is a carbonic anhydrase inhibitor. Acetazolamide decreases the sodium hydrogen ion exchange and increases the excretion of sodium bicarbonate for sodium chloride. Because acetazolamide prevents the regeneration of filtered bicarbonate, a metabolic acidosis can ensue.

C and 2. The loop diuretic furosemide increases the excretion of potassium, magnesium, and calcium.

D and 4. Thiazide diuretics impair glucose tolerance and increase serum lipid levels. The maintenance of a normal serum potassium level attenuates the effect on glucose and lipid metabolism.

87 Abdominal compartment syndrome occurs when the pressure in a confined anatomical space increases to the point where perfusion is compromised. Typically, this condition occurs after traumatic injury and large volumes of fluid resuscitation. Visceral edema is exacerbated by shock-induced hypoperfusion, reperfusion, and mesenteric venous occlusion caused by surgical manipulation. Abdominal compartment hypertension decreases cardiac output by increasing systemic vascular resistance, decreasing venous return, increasing after load, and elevating intrathoracic pressure. Mesenteric blood flow may be decreased to the point of visceral ischemia. Compression of the renal veins also contributes to oliguria. Pulmonary compliance is decreased and peak airway pressures are increased. The exact pressure at which these adverse physiologic effects occur varies, but they can usually be detected when pressures exceed 20 mmHg (2.7 kPa) and become severe when pressures exceed 40 mmHg (5.3 kPa). Intra-abdominal pressures may be reliably approximated by transducing gastric pressures via an nasogastric tube or intravesicular pressures via a foley catheter. Abdominal compartment syndrome can be both avoided and treated by use of a temporary abdominal closure using a prosthetic material (e.g. mesh or an IV fluid bag) sewn to the patient's skin.

88–90: Questions

88 An 85-year-old male with a history of hypertension, COPD, CHF, and gout is brought to the emergency department by his family. Over the last several weeks the patient has had a change in mental status, generalized weakness, anorexia, and diarrhea. ECG shows sinus bradycardia with a rate of 32/min. The patient's symptoms are most consistent with which of the following:
A Theophylline toxicity.
B Beta blocker toxicity.
C Colchicine toxicity.
D Digoxin toxicity.

89 The patient is a 72-year-old male with a nonhealing ulcer over the first metatarsal head plantar surface. His medical history is significant for diabetes and vasculitis. Medications include insulin and prednisone. The patient is afebrile, and has some serous drainage from the 2 × 2 cm (0.8 × 0.8 in) ulcer. Pitting edema is noted on the dorsum of the foot, and there is 5 mm (0.2 in) of paranoid erythema. His ankle brachial index is 0.8. The patient's hemoglobin is 95 g/l (9.5 g/dl), and WBC is 8.0×10^9/l (8,000/mm^3). Which of the following management steps are indicated?
A Vitamin A therapy.
B Vitamin E therapy.
C Leg elevation.
D Vascular bypass.
E Transfusion of U packed cells.
F Immediate incision and drainage.

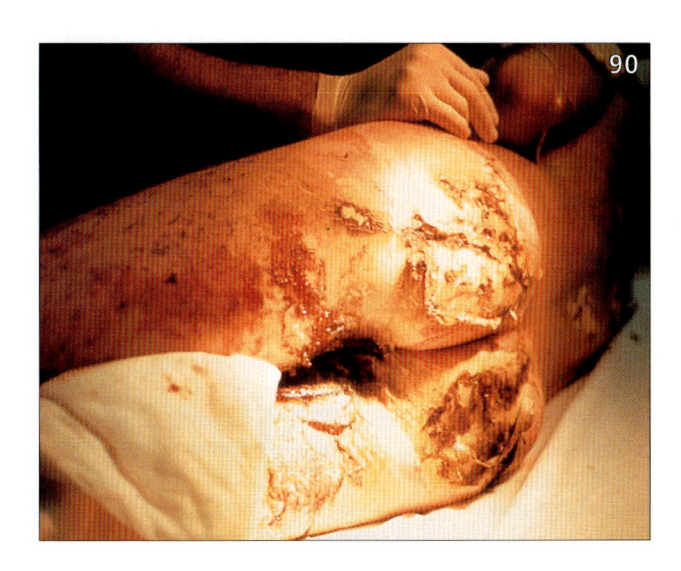

90 This patient (**90**) suffered an extensive electrical burn and is about to undergo debridement. What monitoring lines are needed?

88–90: Answers

88 D. Naturally occurring analogs of digoxin can be found in certain plants including foxglove, oleander, and lily of the valley. It can also present in the skins of certain species of toads. The therapeutic effects of digoxin have been known for centuries. Digoxin inhibits the Na-K ATPase pump in myocardial tissue resulting in increased contractility and decreased AV node conduction. The half-life of digoxin is 36–48 hours and it is eliminated through renal excretion. Toxic manifestations can occur at therapeutic serum levels and conversely, high serum levels do not necessarily indicate toxicity. Clinical correlation with the patient's symptoms is necessary. Toxicity is exacerbated by advanced age, ischemic heart disease, electrolyte disturbances (hypokalemia, hypomagnesemia, and hypercalcemia), and hypoxia. Signs and symptoms of toxicity include anorexia, nausea and vomiting, diarrhea, lightheadedness, weakness, headache, confusion, disorientation, delirium, and seizures. The patient may see yellow-green halos. Any cardiac arrhythmia is possible in toxic states including supraventricular arrhythmias, ventricular arrhythmias, bradyarrhythmias, tachyarrhythmias, and conduction blocks. Treatment involves supportive care and correction of electrolyte abnormalities and arrhythmias. Class 1A antiarrhythmics, procainamide, and quinidine are contraindicated in the treatment of digoxin induced arrhythmias. Cardioversion is also contraindicated as it can lead to intractable ventricular fibrillation. Digoxin specific Fab fragments (Digibind) is expensive and is indicated only for refractory hyperkalemia (K^+ >5.5) and life-threatening ventricular and bradyarrhythmias unresponsive to conventional therapy.

89 A and C. Vitamin A therapy, at 25,000 units/day systemically or topically administered at 50,000 units/ounce of vehicle, will reverse the steroid induced healing impediment. Leg elevation for control of edema is crucial in optimizing cellular perfusion and oxygenation. Vitamin E may retard healing, and more data is required to determine whether vascular bypass would clearly benefit this patient. Cellular oxygenation is adequate with a hemoglobin of 6 g or greater, as long as the cardiopulmonary delivery system is not compromised. This ulcer is not infected, though it is at high risk, and does not need immediate incision and drainage.

90 Electrical burns may be associated with significant, deep, but hidden tissue destruction. Patients may develop combinations of myoglobinuria, hyperkalemia, and, or, renal failure. For this reason, and because this patient will obviously require extensive debridement, a foley catheter and central line are both mandatory. Another issue is the risk of cardiac dysfunction and, or, dysrhythmias. Electrical injuries that appear to have crossed the body (e.g. entering the left hand and exiting the right foot) are obviously associated with the possibility of myocardial damage and instability. This can be assessed preoperatively by echocardiography and ECG. However, in the absence of suspected myocardial dysfunction, pulmonary artery occlusion catheters are not always required, and might be considered a potential source of arythmogensis. Cardiac rhythm should be carefully monitored. Electrolyte abnormalities and acid/base abnormalities should be aggressively corrected.

91–93: Questions

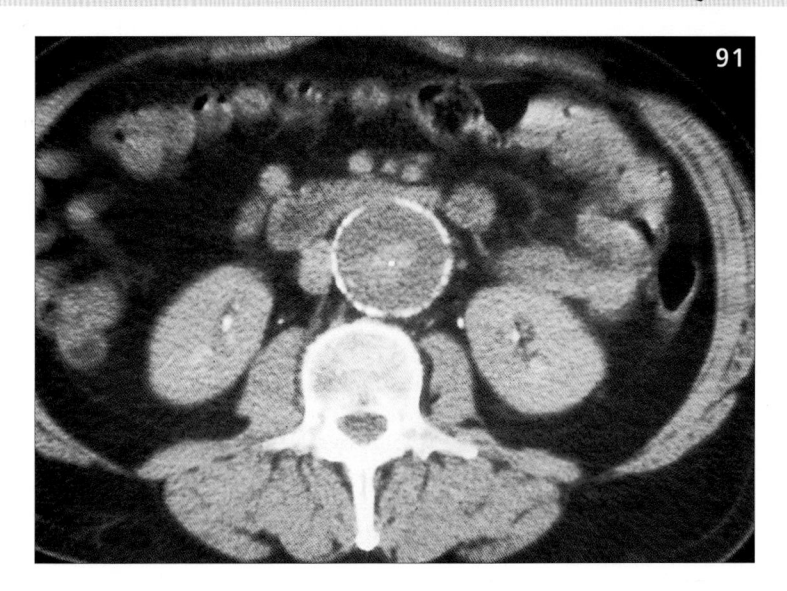

91 A patient being evaluated for acute abdominal pain has an abdominal CT scan performed (**91**). As he is being transferred from the scanner he becomes unresponsive and you can no longer feel a pulse. What pathology does the CT scan demonstrate? What is the next step in this patient's management?

92 A 59-year-old male presents with fever and a productive cough with greenish sputum. Gram stain reveals small Gram-negative rods. Colonies grow on chocolate agar supplemented with heme and NAD^+. What is the causative organism?

93 A 3-year-old female has been admitted to the ICU with suspected epiglottitis. Her condition deteriorates and she requires intubation. What method of inducing anesthesia is appropriate?

91–93: Answers

91 This patient has CT scan findings consistent with abdominal aortic aneurysm. CT has become the gold standard for evaluation of the abdominal aortic aneurysm. Ultrasound is useful for interval surveillance and is less expensive as well as less invasive. However, CT is the most accurate at determining true size of the aneurysm and yields more information concerning proximal and distal involvement. It is also highly accurate at determining rupture. Given the history and clinical state his only hope is emergency operation.

92 *Haemophilus influenzae*.

93 The immediate priority with this patient is control of her airway while avoiding life-threatening airway obstruction. An inhalational induction is mandatory as intravenous agents may cause immediate loss of the airway. This will be impossible to visualize at laryngoscopy because of the swelling caused by the epiglottitis. Inhalational agents by contrast wear off quickly and airway tone is more quickly regained. Any procedure stressful to the child may precipitate complete obstruction. Distress to the child will result in coughing, crying, and obstruction. This includes placement of an intravenous cannula or even performing neck radiographs so these procedures should be avoided. Halothane or sevoflurane are the induction agents of choice. They act quickly and are reasonably pleasant to inhale. Halothane is used in slowly increasing concentrations up to 5% in 100% oxygen. Sevoflurane 8% in 100% can be used immediately as its blood gas solubility is low enough to allow rapid inhalational anesthesia. Induction of anesthesia may take some time with either agent because coughing and airway obstruction may subsequently worsen. These factors can be relieved by placing the child supine, or by application of continuous positive airways pressure via the facemask. As anesthesia deepens, oxygen consumption should reduce and arterial oxygen saturation improve. An intravenous cannula should be sited at this stage and once a plane of surgical anesthesia is reached laryngoscopy is performed and an oral ET is placed. This can be changed at a later date to a nasotracheal tube.

94–96: Questions

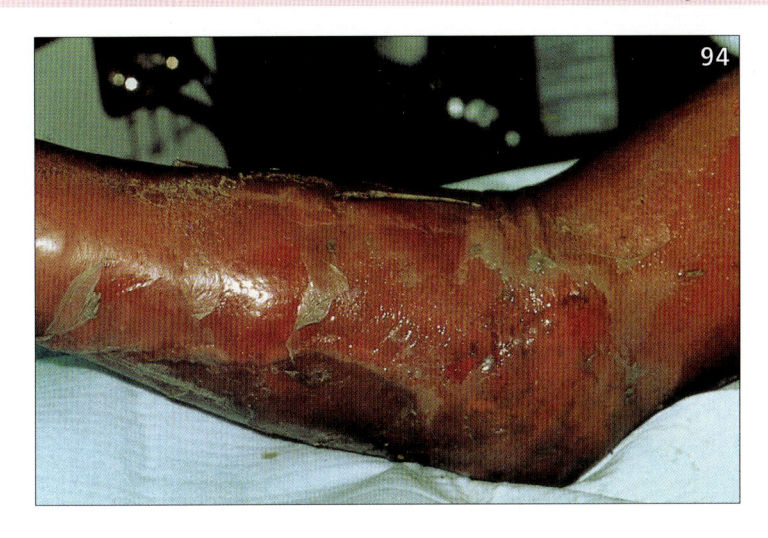

94 How would you manage this patient (**94**)?

95 Match the following Gram-negative bacteria (A–F) with the culture/Gram stain results (1–6).
A *Klebsiella pneumonia.*
B *Neisseria meningitidis.*
C *Legionella pneumophila.*
D *Haemophilus influenzae.*
E *Pseudomonas aeruginosa.*
F *Escherichia coli.*

1 Weakly Gram-negative rods, requires L-cysteine and iron to grow.
2 Small Gram-rods (occasionally reported as cocci initially), requires hematin and NAD$^+$ for growth. Culture on chocolate agar.
3 Gram-negative rods, beta-hemolytic, obligate aerobe, and lactose fermenter.
4 Gram-negative rods, lactose fermenting, and indole negative.
5 Gram-negative rods, obligate aerobe, oxidase positive, and a nonlactose fermenter.
6 Kidney-shaped diplococci, a facultative anaerobe, and ferments glucose and maltose.

96 The drug of choice in refractory status epilepticus is:
A Anesthetic doses of phenobarbital.
B Phenothiazine.
C Diazepam 15 mg IV push.
D Neuromuscular blockade.
E Phenytoin 100 mg/kg IV push.

94–96: Answers

94 i. This patient has a severe soft-tissue infection. A simplified system of classification is based upon the bacterial causative agent of the soft-tissue infection, that being either clostridial or nonclostridial infections. A nonclostridial infection can be a single bacterium infection or an infection with multiple bacteria. The involved tissue can be skin and subcutaneous tissues or skin through to the muscle layers. Principles of management of this lesion include recognizing whether this is a local problem only versus systemic involvement with the infection. An immediate aspiration of fluid from the blisters with Gram stain or tissue Gram stain is performed. The broad antibiotic coverage is guided by the Gram-stain results. The patient with systemic symptoms needs aggressive fluid resuscitation including large caliber intravenous lines, invasive monitoring, and tetanus prophylaxis. Wide surgical debridement is necessary. The debridement must extend to viable tissue and may include amputation. Hyperbaric oxygen therapy may be effective with clostridial infections, but remains unproven in nonclostridial infections. Gamma globulin may be useful in Gram-positive infections.

95 Often therapy must be based on Gram-stain results interpreted in the light of the clinical situation. *Klebsiella pneumonia* (4) is associated with pneumonia and urinary infections. Treatment includes cephalosporins, aminoglycosides and, or, bactrim. *Neisseria meningitidis* (6) is associated with meningitis, sepsis, and Waterhouse–Freidrickson syndrome of hemorrhagic adrenal infarct. Treatment includes penicillin, ceftriaxone, and rifampin prophylaxis. It is a vaccine against capsule antigens A, C, and Y. *Legionella pneumophila* (1) is associated with Legionnaire's disease and pneumonia. Treatment includes erthromycin and, or, rifampin. *Haemophilus influenzae* (2) is encapsulated and is associated with meningitis, pneumonia, sepsis, septic arthritis in infants, and epiglottitis. The rarer nonencapsulated form is associated with otitis media and sinusitis. Treatment includes ampicillin and cephalosporins. *Pseudomonas aeruginosa* (5) is associated with several virulent conditions including pneumonia (especially in cystic fibrosis and immuno-compromised patients), osteomyelitis (especially diabetics and IV drug abusers), burn wound sepsis, urinary infections, endocarditis, and corneal infections in contact lens wearers. Treatment includes penicillins and aminoglycosides. *Escherichia coli* (3) is associated with intrabdominal sepsis, newborn meningitis, nosocomial sepsis, pneumonia, and diarrhea. Treatment includes metronidazole, penicillins, and cephalosporins.

96 A. Phenothiazines and neuromuscular blockade play no role in treatment of status epilepticus. Diazepam and phenytoin are first and second line drugs while high doses of phenobarbital or pentobarbital are the drugs of choice when the condition is unresponsive to benzodiazepines and phenytoin. Ventilatory assistance and vasopressors are always necessary at this point. Diazepam and paraldehyde can be given rectally.

97–99: Questions

97 A 47-year-old female was found unresponsive in her hospital bed 2 days after having had a total hip arthroplasty under epidural anesthesia. Her vital signs are: BP 75/40 mmHg (10.0/5.3 kPa), HR 120/min, and RR 38/min. Her past medical history is significant for rheumatoid arthritis for which she took nonsteroidal anti-inflammatory medications and glucocorticosteriods. She has had a previous cervical fusion at C1–C2. Preoperative flexion–extension views of the cervical spine are shown (**97a, b**).

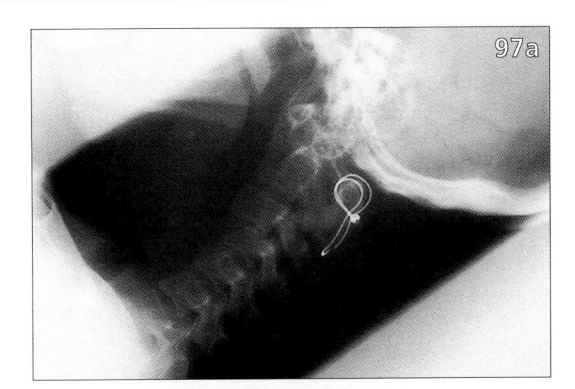

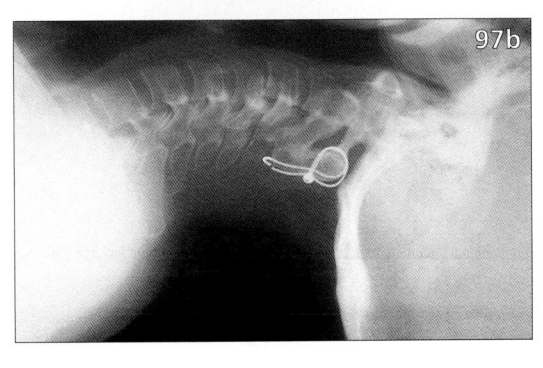

The patient is stabilized with oxygen by bag-valve-mask and preparations are made to intubate. Which one of the following is most appropriate?
A Blind nasotracheal intubation with cervical stabilization in a flexed position.
B Direct laryngoscopy and oral intubation with cervical stabilization in a flexed position.
C Direct laryngoscopy and oral intubation with cervical stabilization in a neutral position.
D Fiberoptic nasotracheal intubation with cervical stabilization in a neutral position.

98 The major systemic derangement caused by status epilepticus includes all of the following except:
A Hypoxia.
B Hyperglycemia.
C Hyperthermia.
D Acidosis.
E Hypotension.

99 A 100 kg (222 lb) patient comes to the ICU after an emergency total abdominal colectomy for lower gastrointestinal bleeding. His vital signs are normal: the CVP is 5.0 mmHg (0.7 kPa) and the urine output is 30 ml/hr. How do you evaluate this low urine output?

97–99: Answers

97 C. This patient has severe arthritic changes in her cervical spine with atlantoaxial instability despite a previous fusion, as well as C3–C4 subluxation. Manipulation of the cervical spine into extreme flexion or extension may result in severe spinal cord injury. In an emergency situation, direct laryngoscopy with oral intubation is the most appropriate means of securing the airway. Where cervical spine pathology coexists with a compromised airway, emergent management includes stabilization of the cervical spine in a neutral position while intubation is accomplished. Fiberoptic intubation should be reserved for more elective situations.

98 B. All of the above are true except for hyperglycemia. Status can cause hypoglycemia, placing the brain at risk. Serum glucose levels must be closely monitored.

99 This patient is oliguric, that is the urine output is <0.5 ml/kg/hr. Prerenal, renal parenchyma dysfunction, and postrenal dysfunction must be evaluated in this patient. The CVP is 5.0 mmHg (0.7 kPa) in this patient and denotes diminished intravascular volume. Volume status and urine examination are evaluated below. Nephrotoxic drugs must be discontinued. Postrenal dysfunction with evaluation of the collecting system by ultrasonography, intravenous pyelogram or a cystourethrogram can be performed. In the circumstance of a pelvic operation, there is concern regarding ligation of the ureter. If this is the cause of the oliguria, the patient must be re-explored. Both ureters are examined and repaired if necessary. Prerenal dysfunction causes 50–90% of the total cases of acute renal failure. Renal parenchymal dysfunction is related to 10–30% of total cases. Postrenal dysfunction is related to 1–15% of cases.

Urine output <0.5 ml/kg/hr

Prerenal	Renal	Postrenal
Volume status Renal artery function Renogram	Volume status Stop toxic drugs	Volume status Intravenous pyelogram/ultrasound
High specific gravity pH <6 Urine Na^+ <20 $FeNa^+$ <2 Hyaline cast	Low specific gravity Urine Na^+ >40 $FeNa^+$ >1 Casts – multiple types	Normal specific gravity pH 6 Urine Na^+ >40 $FeNa^+$ >3
Maintain volume Repair artery	Maintain volume Role diuretic/low dose dopamine Evaluate dialysis	Bladder catheter Suprapubic catheter Nephrostomy Repair ureter

100, 101: Questions

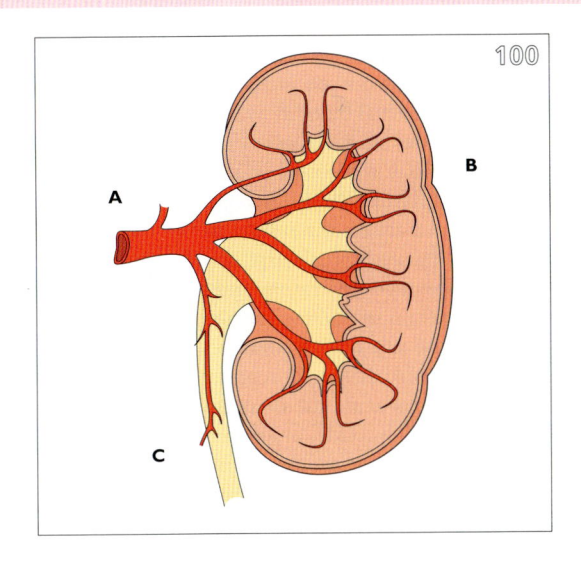

100 Match the area of kidney pathology (**100, A, B, C**) to the profile below.

	Profile 1	Profile 2
Urine Na⁺ (mmol/l) (mEq/l)	>40	<20
Urine/plasma creatinine (mmol/l) (mg/dl)	<1,770 (<20)	>3,540 (>40)
Urine osmolality (mOsm/kg)	<350	>500
Urine/plasma osmolality (mOsm/kg)	1.0	>1.2
Fractional excretion of sodium (%)	>1	<1
Renal failure index (%)	>1	<1
Free water clearance (ml/hr)	Positive	Negative

101 A 20-year-old female is being cared for in the ICU following a pedestrian accident. She was hit by a motor vehicle and sustained a mild closed head injury, pulmonary contusion requiring intubation and ventilation, left arm fracture, and right femoral fracture requiring internal fixation and stabilization. Three days after admission, she experiences a worsening of her pulmonary condition and spikes a temperature of 39°C (102.2°F) and has mild abdominal distension with increased nasogastric tube output. Before her orthopedic operation, she had a negative diagnostic peritoneal lavage. Serum amylase and WBC counts are increasing. What are the causes of serum amylase increase after blunt trauma in this patient? What would you do?

100, 101: Answers

100 Area A matches with profile 2. This area represents prerenal causes of acute renal failure where there is a significant decline in renal blood flow. Because the glomerular filtration rate is dependent upon renal blood flow, the glomerular filtration rate decreases. The etiology for prerenal causes of acute renal failure includes a decrease in cardiac output, hypotension, hepatorenal syndrome, bilateral renal artery stenosis, and angiotensin converting enzyme inhibitors, NSAIDs, and cyclosporin. The urinalysis shows traces of protein and hyalin casts. As the tubule in the tubular network is intact, the kidney responds to prerenal causes by reabsorption of sodium and water. The resulting urine typically has a low sodium concentration and a high osmolarity. The renal failure index and the fractional excretion of sodium are normal. When net water reabsorption occurs, the free water clearance is a negative number indicating tubular reabsorption of water. Area B matches with profile 1. Area B represents intrarenal or structural causes of acute renal failure which includes acute tubule necrosis from nephrotoxic agents. These agents include antibiotics (aminoglycoside, amphotericin, penicillin, and cephalosporins), heavy metal toxicity, radiographic contrast agents, myoglobin, hemoglobin, and myeloma chains. Patients with acute tubule necrosis have an active urine sediment which shows granular casts and sloughed renal tubular cells. Because the tubular network is not intact, sodium concentration is generally >40 mmol/l (mEq/l) and the urine is isotonic. The fractional excretion of sodium in the renal failure index is generally greater than three. Since there is a failure to concentrate the urine, the free water clearance is positive. Area C represents postrenal insults which include bladder obstruction or bilateral ureter obstruction either from stones, cancer, or strictures.

101 Amylase elevation can occur after trauma from injury to face and salivary glands, injury to stomach, small bowel, and pancreas. An elevation in serum amylase is not by itself an indication for exploratory laparotomy, but when accompanied by a positive physical examination, pancreatic or bowel injury is likely. Trauma to the pancreas occurs in approximately 1.4% of all injuries related to blunt abdominal trauma. Contusion, transection, and pseudocyst formation can all occur. Because the pancreas is a retroperitoneal organ, diagnostic peritoneal lavage is not helpful in making the diagnosis of this injury. The patient may present with mild upper abdominal tenderness and minimal other signs of injury. A CT scan of the abdomen is helpful in defining injury to the pancreas if the scan is delayed by 12–24 hours. This delay allows hematoma and swelling to take place just around the pancreas. The CT can identify parenchymal disruption, diffuse enlargement, parapancreatic fluid collections, or pseudocysts (**101**). This injury is very difficult to identify in the absence of other intra-abdominal organ injuries and diagnosis is often delayed.

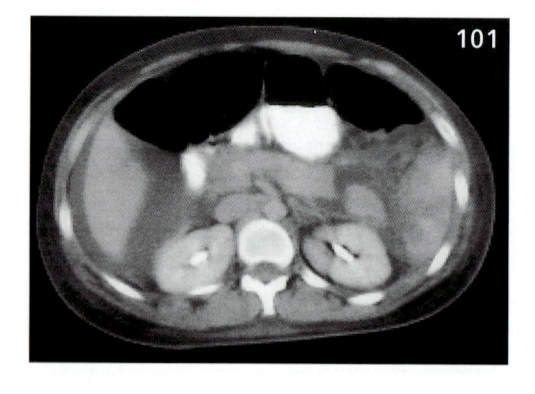

102–104: Questions

102 A 4-year-old male presents to the emergency department with his father. The child was playing in the yard and was later found in the garage with watery eyes and frothing at the mouth. His vital signs are temperature 36.8°C (98.2°F), pulse 58/min, BP 90/60 mmHg (12.0/8.0 kPa), and RR 12/min. The symptoms are most consistent with:
A Rat poisoning.
B Pesticide poisoning.
C Hydrocarbon poisoning.
D Mercury poisoning.

103 In the last 20 years, survival rates following major burns have improved to the point where there is no median lethal dose with respect to burn size in young children. This has been attributed predominantly to the practice of early excision and grafting of burns. How does this practice contribute to greater survival rates?

104 Based on the energy cycle presented (**104**), discuss the following:
i. Differences between anaerobic and aerobic metabolism.
ii. The implication of lactate/pyruvate ratio.

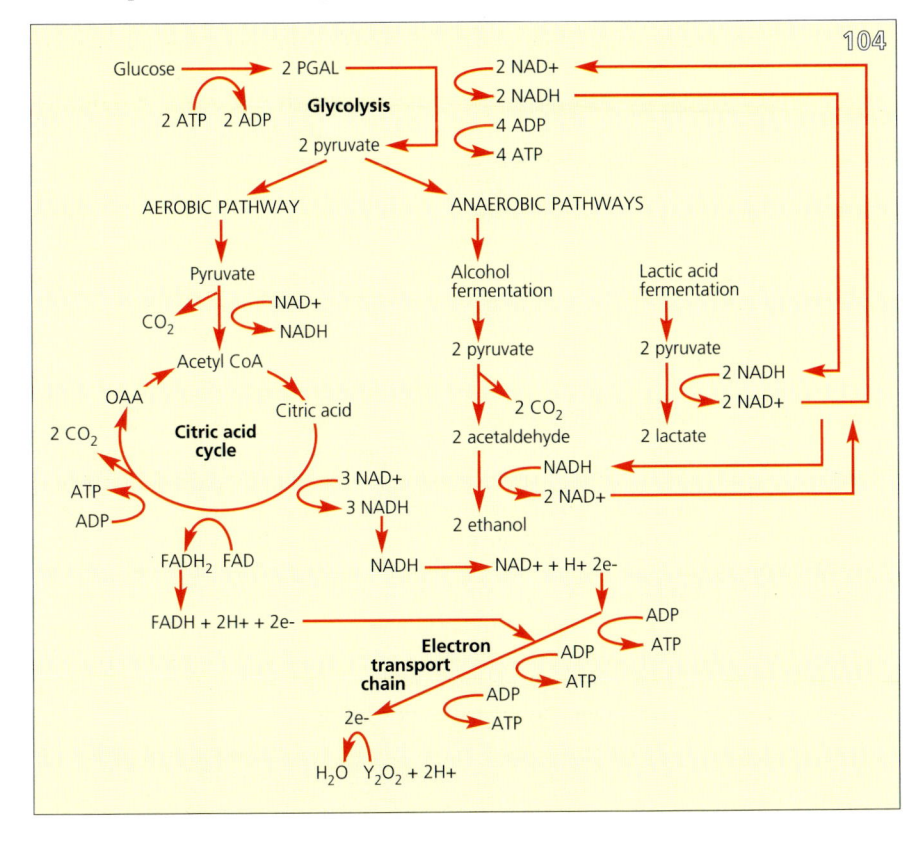

102–104: Answers

102 B. Most insecticides contain OPs. OP insecticides are popular for both agricultural and home use because their unstable chemical structure leads to rapid hydrolysis into harmless compounds. OPs, however, are highly toxic. They irreversibly bind to cholinesterase molecules and permanently inactive them. The inhibition of cholinesterase activity leads to excess accumulation of acetylcholine at nerve synapses. All receptors are affected including central, peripheral, nicotinic, and muscarinic. OPs can be absorbed by oral, dermal, conjunctival, gastrointestinal, and respiratory routes. Clinical manifestations can occur immediately or can be delayed by as much as 24 hours depending on the route of contamination. Muscarinic overstimulation leads to hyperactivity of the parasympathetic nervous system. Nicotinic effects include muscle fasciculation, cramping, and weakness. CNS manifestations include delirium, confusion, coma, seizures, and respiratory depression. Diagnosis is usually made on clinical grounds. Decreased serum and RBC cholinesterase activity can be measured, but the laboratory results will not be readily available in the acute setting. Treatment involves aggressive airway management for secretions, pulmonary edema, respiratory depression, and muscle weakness. IV atropine should be administered. The dose is 2 mg every 5–15 minutes in adults and 0.05 mg/kg every 15 minutes in children as necessary until atropinization (mydriasis, tachycardia, flushing, and drying of secretions) is established. Pralidoxime is a biochemical antidote for OP poisoning that can reverse the cholinergic nicotinic effects. It should be given within 24–36 hours of exposure and only used for symptomatic patients. Ventricular arrhythmias can occur with organophosphate poisoning and can be treated with lidocaine, bretylium, cardioversion, isoproterenol hydrochloride, or overdrive pacing.

103 Early excision and grafting (within the first 5 days after injury) removes the infectious and metabolic load resulting from an open skin envelope. Removal of devitalized tissue decreases the amount of bacteria that has direct access to the blood stream. It also decreases the loss of heat, protein, and fluids out of the open wound. Early excision and grafting is the engine behind the majority of progress made in survival rates after major burns.

104 i. Aerobic metabolism implies respiration in the presence of oxygen and includes glycolysis, the citric acid cycle, and oxidative phosphorylation. Anaerobic metabolism is a form of fermentation in which stores of phosphocreatinine and glycogen are used to generate ATP with lactate being a byproduct. The ratio of glucose utilized to ATP produced in aerobic respiration is 2:36 while it is only 2:2 for anaerobic, which is much less efficient.

ii. The normal lactate/pyruvate ratio is <10:1. Normal arterial lactate is 0.5–1.6 mmol/l (mEq/l) and pyruvate 0.03–0.1 mmol/l (mEq/l). Increases in the lactate/pyruvate ratio imply anaerobic conditions. Because pyruvate is very unstable when withdrawn, and because conditions such as increased glycolysis can increase the lactate/pyruvate ratio in the absence of ischemia, this ratio has limited clinical utility.

105, 106: Questions

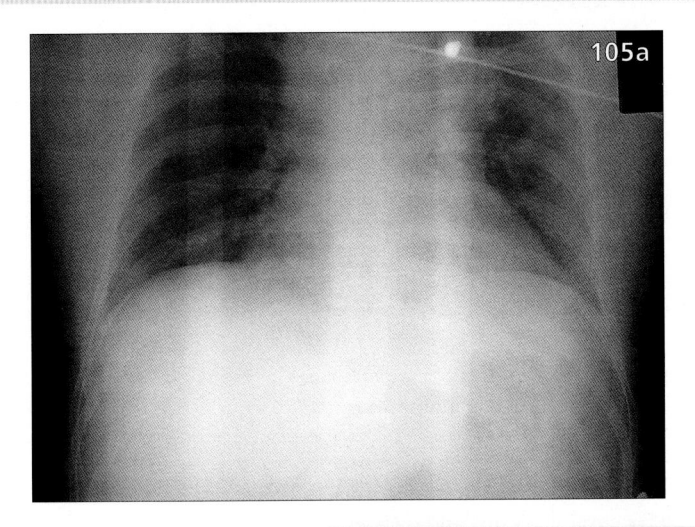

105 A 36-year-old construction worker suffered a torso crush injury in a crane arm accident. A left chest needle thoracostomy was performed by the helicopter transport team for diminished left chest breath sounds with relief of pneumothorax. Initial vital signs included a pulse of 125/min, a systolic BP of 110 mmHg (14.7 kPa) and a RR 40/min. The patient had abdominal tenderness. The initial chest X-ray is shown (**105a**).
i. What diagnosis is suggested by the chest X-ray? What other chest X-ray findings would suggest the same diagnosis? What should be the next diagnostic step? What other procedures should be performed?
ii. The patient also underwent diagnostic peritoneal lavage which was grossly positive. At laparotomy, a grade IV liver laceration was found. Given the aortogram findings shown here (**105b**), how should the necessary operative procedures be sequenced and why?

106 You are evaluating a 24-year-old male who was in a significant motor vehicle crash. As you are examining him you notice that he is able to speak but that the words are inappropriate and he is clearly disoriented. He does appear to localize pain but is unable to follow commands. His eyes only open to severe pain. What is his Glasgow coma score and how is it determined?

105, 106: Answers

105 i. Mediastinal widening is the hallmark of aortic and, or, great vessel injury. Other signs include: first rib, scapula, or clavicle fracture; left hemothorax or apical cap; loss of aortic knob or anteroposterior projection window; deviation of the nasogastric or endotracheal tube; and left mainstem bronchus depression. Aortography is the diagnostic modality of choice for diagnosis and therapeutic planning for aortic and great vessel injury. Transesophageal echo may have a role in diagnosis for patients with need for life-saving laparotomy, but does have a significant rate of equivocal findings and there have been false-negative examinations. Spiral chest CT is a newer modality currently being evaluated and may speed the diagnosis in centers with personnel trained in this technique. This patient needs a thorough primary, secondary, and tertiary survey as well as plain radiographs of the cervical spine and pelvis. A diagnostic peritoneal lavage is also indicated.

ii. When faced with combined innominate artery, and severe liver injuries, operative sequence is important. In this case, the liver injury was addressed first with a suture hepatography and packing. No major vascular injuries requiring repair were found. The abdomen was towel-clipped closed during the median sternotomy/vascular repair using partial occlusion clamps and dacron aortic-innominate artery bypass. Systemic anticoagulation (not used in this case) may be necessary, especially in cases requiring atriofemoral or complete cardiopulmonary bypass and necessitates close communication between the surgical teams.

106 The Glasgow coma scale was developed to assess level of consciousness. It is scored from 3–15 with three contributing components. Best response from each category is evaluated and scored by a standard scale (see below). Generally a score of 8 or less means the patient is in a coma. Changes in the Glasgow coma score of 2–3 are generally significant and suggest enlarging hematoma. The Glasgow coma score is unreliable in patients with alcohol or other drugs in their systems, and patients who are hypotensive.

Eye opening		Best motor response		Best verbal response	
Spontaneous	4	Follows commands	6	Oriented	5
To voice	3	Localizes	5	Disoriented	4
To pain	2	Flexion withdrawal	4	Inappropriate words	3
None	1	Abnormal flexion	3	Sounds only	2
		Extension	2	None	1
		None	1		

This patient scored 2 for eye opening, 5 for best motor response, and 3 for best verbal response. His total Glasgow coma score is 10.

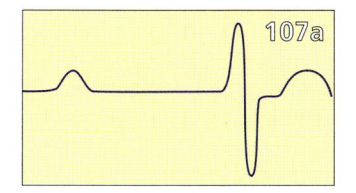

107–109: Questions

107 Diagnose the following forms of heart block (**107a–d**).

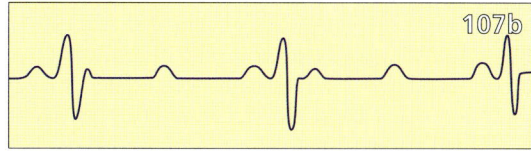

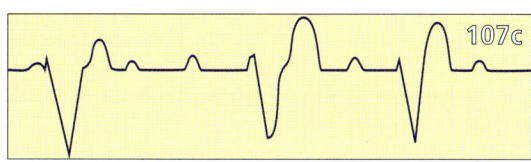

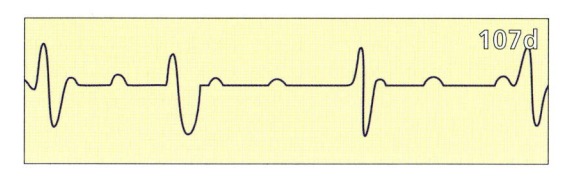

108 A 56-year-old male was involved with a fire in his home (**108**). He was found in a smoke filled room. He has 30% second degree body surface area burns. He is coughing and complains of a sore throat. His coughing produces a carbonatious sputum. Examination reveals increasing wheezing. The next best step in the workup is:
A ABGs.
B Epinephrine.
C Chest X-ray.
D Hyperbaric oxygen.
E Bronchoscopy.

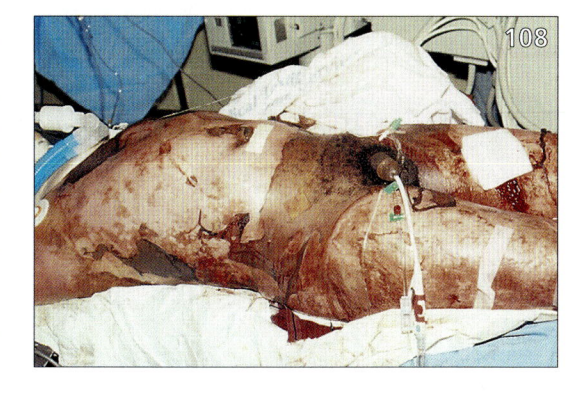

109 Which statement is true regarding inhalation anesthesia for refractory status epilepticus?
A Halothane is superior to isoflurane for suppressing seizures.
B Renal toxicity is a complication of halothane.
C Isoflurane is associated with significant hemodynamic side effects.
D Isoflurane is not hepatotoxic at doses required to suppress seizure activity.
E Halothane suppresses seizures by increasing intracellular magnesium.

107–109: Answers

107 (**107a**). First degree (prolonged P–R); (**107b**). Moblitz type II second degree block (intermittently transmitted P waves); (**107c**). Complete, third degree, heart block (unrelated P waves with wide idioventricular rhythm); (**107d**). Moblitz type I (Wenkebach), second degree block (progressively longer P–R until the atrial impulse is blocked at the A–V node).

108 D. Smoke inhalation should be suspected. Immediate management includes the application of humidified oxygen, controlled fluid intake (two-thirds of the calculated requirements) and an urgent assessment of the airway. If the patient has gross stridor or other obvious signs of airway distress, immediate intubation should be performed as the airway edema can increase rapidly and cause loss of the airway. If there are only mild signs or symptoms, bronchoscopy or fiberoptic laryngoscopy can be performed to confirm upper airway edema and provide an avenue for intubation. There is no evidence that prophylactic antibiotics or steroids are helpful in these patients. The pathophysiology of smoke inhalation involves both heat trauma and inhaled substances, notably carbon monoxide. Signs and symptoms of carbon monoxide poisoning include confusion, headache, and cardiovascular collapse. Blood gases will reveal the presence of carboxyhemoglobin. Signs and symptoms of confusion usually indicate levels >15%. Levels of 60% or greater are usually fatal. The treatment of carbon monoxide poisoning is 100% oxygen. The half-life of carboxyhemoglobin is 90 minutes in room air, approximately 30 minutes on 100% oxygen, and is much quicker in hyperbaric oxygen at three atmospheres. Although hyperbaric oxygenation is recommended in stable patients with evidence of carbon monoxide poisoning, its overall utility is controversial.

109 D. Isoflurane is a superior inhalation agent over halothane. Halothane can cause hepatotoxicity and hemodynamic side effects. Halothane does not suppress seizures by increasing intracellular magnesium. Isoflurane anesthesia is recommended for a small subgroup of patients in status epilepticus who have advanced liver disease and in whom phenobarbital or pentobarbital anesthesia would be contraindicated.

110–112: Questions

110 A 58-year-old patient is admitted to the hospital with a diagnosis of acute pancreatitis. He denies any history of alcohol intake or use of medication. He is febrile (38.6°C/101.5°F), tachycardic and hypotensive. The abdominal examination shows diffuse tenderness, with rebound and guarding. The initial laboratory studies are shown. The ultrasonography study obtained in the emergency room reveals a distended gallbladder with gallstones but without common bile dilation or bile duct calculi; the pancreas could not be visualized due to overlying bowel gas.

> WBC 18.6×10^9/l (18,600/mm^3)
> Glucose 16.81 mmol/l (303 mg/dl)
> Serum glutamic-oxaloacetic transaminase (aspartate transaminase) 288 u/l
> Bilirubin 70.11 μmol/l (4.1 mg/dl)
> Lactic dehydrogenase 1,787 u/l

i. What is your next step?
ii. When would you undertake surgery?

111 Which organism is a common cause of diarrhea, urinary tract infections, meningitis, and septicemia? It has facultative Gram-negative rods and forms lactose fermenting colonies on eosin/methylene blue or MacConkey's agar.

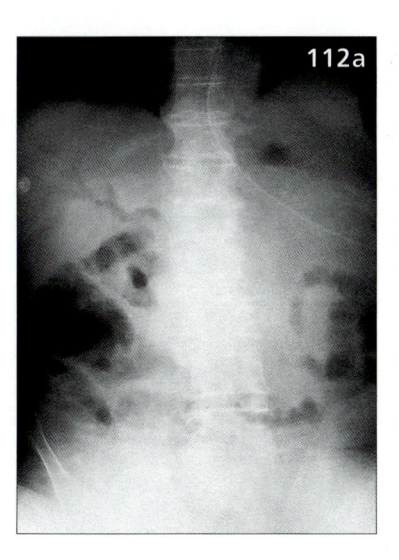

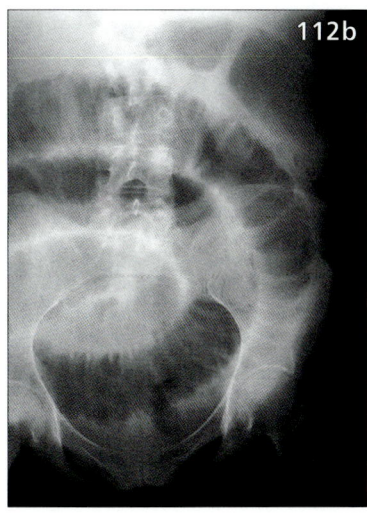

112 A 75-year-old female presents with a 3-day history of bowel obstruction. Abdominal radiographs are taken (**112a, b**). She has a fever and an elevated WBC count. What is your diagnosis?

110–112: Answers

110 i. This patient presents with gallstone pancreatitis. The absence of bile duct stones on the initial imaging study does not rule out the presence of calculi, because most stones inducing acute pancreatitis tend to be small and ultrasonography is an insensitive method to search for choledocholithiasis. The initial step in the treatment of patients with acute pancreatitis is the clinical evaluation and stratification using clinical or serologic markers to distinguish edematous forms of the disease, which tend to be mild, versus necrotizing pancreatitis carrying a mortality of 20–40%. This patient had four positive Ranson's criteria, associated with an increased risk of morbidity and mortality. The next step should be to obtain a CT scan of the abdomen and evaluate the extent of tissue necrosis. The extent of necrosis is linked closely with the outcome of the patient.

ii. Biliary surgery in patients with severe gallstone pancreatitis should be deferred until the patient is stabilized. Biliary decompression in such cases can be achieved using urgent endoscopic-retrograde cholangiography with sphincterotomy and stone removal. However, the role of endoscopic-retrograde cholangiography in patients with acute pancreatitis shows only a clear benefit in the subgroup of patients who present with cholangitis, ductal obstruction, and a failure to clinically improve.

111 *Escherichia coli*.

112 These abdominal films are compatible with gallstone ileus. Air is seen in the biliary tree along with small bowel obstruction. The gallstone has eroded from the gallbladder into the gastrointestinal tract and obstructed it. Two areas which are vulnerable to obstruction are at the ileum 2 cm (0.8 in) in front of the ileocecal valve and the sigmoid colon. These are the two narrowest areas of the bowel. After resuscitation with IV fluids and antibiotics, exploratory laparotomy is indicated. The obstructing gallstone is seen (**112c, d**) and is removed through an enterotomy. There is controversy in the surgical literature about treatment of the biliary-enteric fistula. Repair of this fistula depends on the stability of the patient. If the biliary-enteric fistula is not removed, this patient will be at risk for ascending cholangitis in the future.

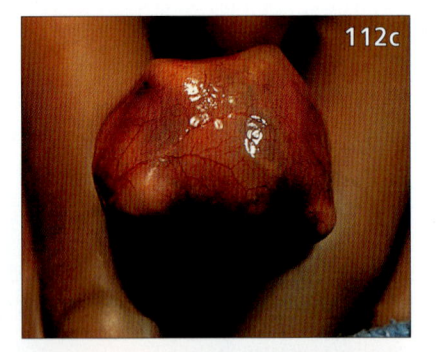

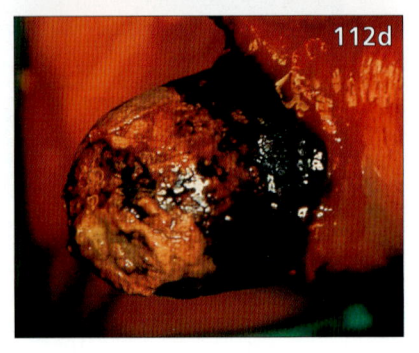

113–116: Questions

113 A 61-year-old male has been admitted to ICU with respiratory distress secondary to an exacerbation of COPD. He is profoundly hypoxic and is close to respiratory arrest. What method of induction of anesthesia is preferable for this patient and why?

114 A 75-year-old bedridden patient develops a fever and a very painful cellulitis on his buttock. The skin appears necrotic and is crepitus. A Gram stain of the exudate shows large Gram-positive rods. What is the causative organism?

115 A 66-year-old male is admitted with right upper quadrant pain, fever, elevated WBC count, and elevated bilirubin. He had endoscopic papillotomy for common duct stones 3 months before this admission. A repeat endoscopic retrograde cholangiography was performed and is shown (**115**). What would you advise?

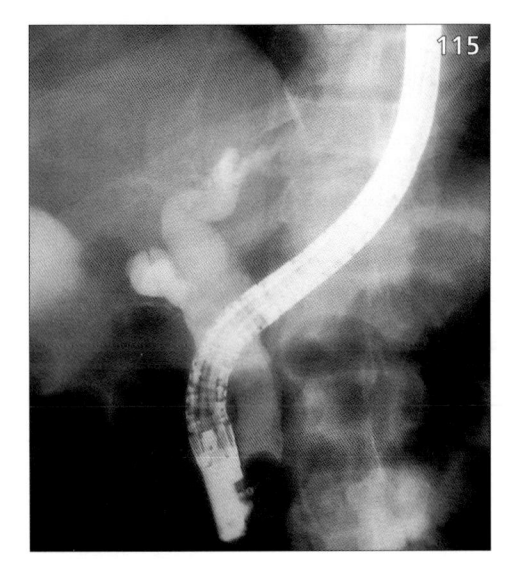

116 Which of the following are true following myocardial infarction?
A A type I (Wenkebach) block requires a temporary pacemaker.
B A type II (Moblitz) block requires a temporary pacemaker.
C Prognosis is worse with anterior myocardial infarction compared to inferior myocardial infarction.
D Premature ventricular contractions (PVCs) are treated by lidocaine routinely.
E Hospital mortality is greater with non-Q wave myocardial infarction.
F Recurrent ischemia is higher with non-Q wave myocardial infarction.
G Post myocardial infarction angina, inability to perform stress test, and persistent ST depression are all risk factors for increased mortality.
H Nitrates decrease mortality following myocardial infarction.
I Nitrates are a first line therapy for angina pectoris.
J Diabetic patients who experience a myocardial infarction have higher mortality than nondiabetics.

113–116: Answers

113 i. Rapid sequence intravenous induction is the technique of choice for this patient. The man has a potential full stomach and severe respiratory distress. It should be possible to either turn the patient or place the patient head down with adequate suction to hand. Cricoid pressure should be used. Bradycardia, due to hypoxia, succinylcholine use, and anesthetic drugs, is likely so atropine and cardiac arrest drugs should be nearby. A precalculated dose of induction agent, e.g. thiopentone at a dose of 3–5 mg/kg or etomidate 0.1–0.2 mg/kg would be suitable. Thiopentone is an effective vasodilator and myocardial depressant and can cause circulatory arrest under circumstances of shock. Etomidate my be a better choice for induction as it confers greater cardiovascular stability. Propofol is best avoided due to its known hypotensive effects. The patient may well be dehydrated and the induction dose is, therefore, reduced to prevent sudden and potentially irrecoverable BP drop. Preoxygenation is performed as much as is possible. A tightly applied mask should be used. The induction agent is immediately followed with a dose of 1–2 mg/kg of succinylcholine for paralysis. Drugs are given intravenously in rapid sequence without waiting for effects to occur. The cricoid pressure is maintained for long enough to enable intubation of the trachea *and* the inflation of the cuff. The airway is not protected until the cuff is inflated. Once the airway is secured the chest is auscultated over both lung fields including axillae and over the stomach to rule out esophageal intubation. Once the position of the tube is verified the assistant removes cricoid pressure only.

114 *Clostridium perfringens.*

115 This endoscopic retrograde cholangiography demonstrates a common duct stone. If the stone can be retrieved by endoscopic retrograde cholangiography this should be attempted. If this is successful either laparoscopic or open cholecystectomy should be offered to the patient. If endoscopic retrieval of the stone is not possible, the patient should be prepared for an open cholecystectomy and common bile duct exploration.

116 True: B, C, F, G, I, and J.

117, 118: Questions

117 A 72-year-old male presents to a peripheral hospital with an acute inferior myocardial infarction, his chest pain having begun 36 hours before admission. He was given streptokinase at the community hospital but continues to have ongoing severe pain, ST segment elevation, and evidence of pulmonary edema. He is transferred to your institution where he is found to have a pansystolic apical murmur, evidence of cardiogenic shock, and continued ST elevation, which leads to t-PA administration. A pulmonary artery catheter is inserted and the following determinations are made:

	PO_2 *(mmHg (kPa))*	pH	FiO_2
Systemic	459 (61.2)	7.25	1.0
Pulmonary	78 (10.4)	7.17	1.0
Right atrial	56 (7.5)	7.18	1.0

Discuss the indications for, and outcome of, surgery as well as factors which influence survival.

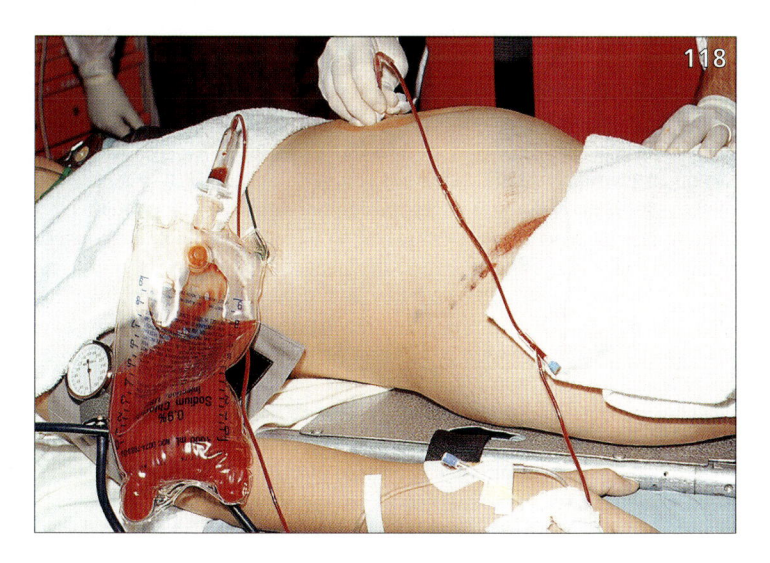

118 A 26-year-old female (**118**), who is in her second trimester of pregnancy, is involved in a motor vehicle crash.
i. What are the anesthetic considerations?
ii. What tests can predict the chance of early labor starting?

117, 118: Answers

117 The data reveal an oxygen step up beyond the right atrium. In this setting the diagnosis of postinfarct ventricular septal rupture is confirmed. Echocardiography (**117**) can also make the diagnosis, but is generally more logistically difficult to obtain. Generally, the presence of such a lesion is an indication for surgery, particularly if severe end organ failure is not present. Without surgery 25% will die in 24 hours and 70% within 2 weeks. Preoperative interval correlates with increasing incidence of multiorgan dysfunction. Only those with small shunts (Qp:Qs<2:1) with very stable hemodynamics should be considered for delayed surgery. Inferior location, right ventricular infarction (common in inferior septal ruptures), elevated right atrial pressure, presence of cardiogenic shock, increasing age, and early rupture following myocardial infarction all have a negative influence on survival. Mortality for anterior defects is in the range of 20–50% and for inferior defects 30–80%, usually closer to the latter. Thrombolytic therapy is suspected of increasing the incidence of all forms of postinfarction myocardial rupture.

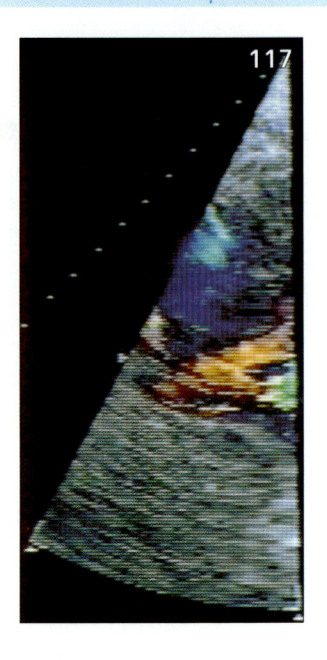

118 i. The primary principle of treating a pregnant patient is to concentrate initially on the mother. There are a number of physiologic responses to pregnancy that need to be taken into account. Mean arterial pressure decreases 5–10 mmHg (0.7–1.3 kPa) during the middle portion of pregnancy. Fluid retention results in a 'dilutional' anemia. This hypervolemia of pregnancy can also result in the masking of significant blood loss. The pregnant uterus can compress the inferior vena cava, and so patients should be positioned with the right side slightly elevated. The upward displacement of the diaphragm results in a reduction of the functional residual capacity by 20%. This leads to a physiologic hyperventilation with normal $PaCO_2$ running at about 30 mmHg (4.0 kPa). Hypoventilation leading to a 'normal' PCO_2 can actually be associated with a relatively significant acidosis. Decreased gastric motility, increased intra-abdominal pressure, and weaker lower esophageal sphincter tone all result in an increased risk of aspiration. Intraoperatively care must be taken not to over ventilate patients, resulting in induction of uterine contractions, nor to hypoventilate patients resulting in decreased placental flow. Alpha-adrenergic agents are associated with decreased placental blood flow and should be avoided if possible.
ii. The risk of fetal death is increased if there is direct uterine injury, maternal shock, pelvic fractures, severe head injuries (Glasgow coma score <9), and admission hypoxia. Non-invasive monitoring, including assessment of fetal heart tones, does not appear sufficiently reliable to be clinically useful to predict the risk of fetal loss. Kleihauer–Betke smears, which detect fetal blood in maternal samples, may provide evidence of placental trauma and be indicative of increased risk of fetal loss.

119–122: Questions

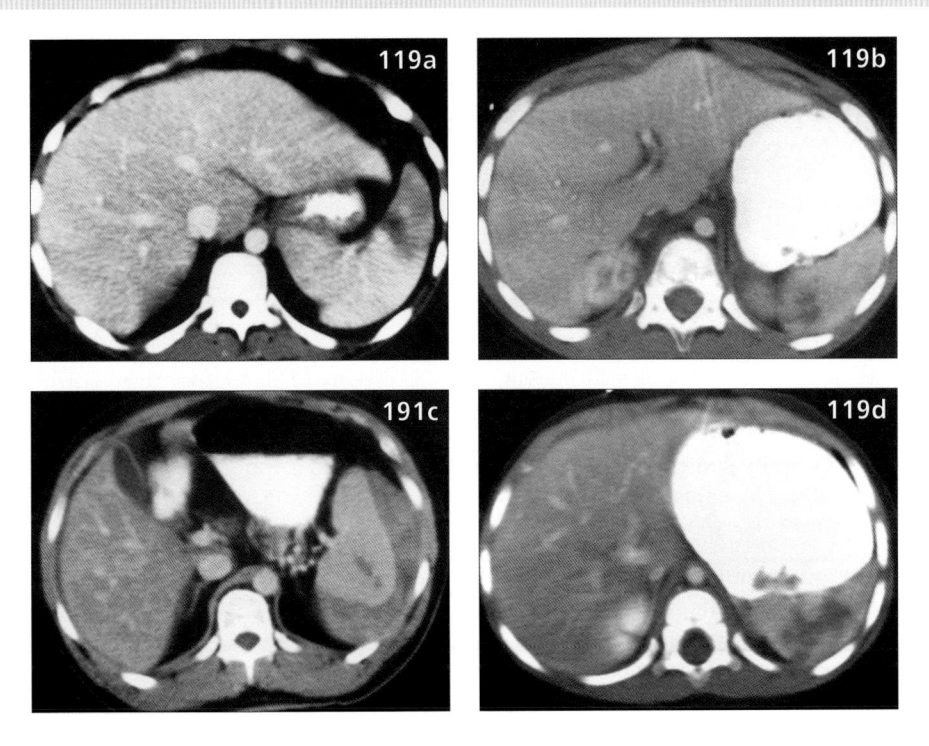

119 Correlate the CT findings (**119a–d**) with the grade of splenic injury.

120 Describe the presentation of acute epiglottitis in a 1-year-old male, 4-year-old male, and a 23-year-old male.

121 A 32-year-old male with a history of IV drug use presents with a fever, fatigue, and a new heart murmur. A blood culture shows Gram-positive cocci in clusters that are beta-hemolytic and coagulase-positive. What is the likely causative organism?

122 A decrease in pulmonary capillary wedge pressure is seen with which of the following agents:
A Epinephrine (adrenaline).
B Isuprel (isoprenaline).
C Dobutamine.
D Dopamine.
E Amrinone hydrochloride.

119–122: Answers

119 The radiologic grading attempts to correlate with the pathologic grading of injury based on the size of laceration or hematoma as well as location. Often, the amount of fluid in the abdomen sways the interpretation. Some centers, when nonoperative management of splenic injuries is employed, will repeat the CT scan to determine whether or not there is increasing amount of peritoneal fluid consistent with ongoing bleeding.
119a Grade I.
119b Grade II.
119c Grade III.
119d Grade IV.

120 The 4-year-old male will present with rapid onset of respiratory distress with stridor, fever (39–40°C/102.2–104°F), and a toxic appearance. The child sits up with head extended, drools, and speaks with a muffled voice. The child has been ill less than 24 hours and coughing is rare. Children less than 24 months of age present atypically. Coughing is present in 50% and most are not toxic appearing. Few children in this group prefer the sitting position and most have a normal voice. Drooling is present in only 50% and 25% are afebrile. Adults usually present 1–2 days after onset of illness with one third presenting at least 4 days after symptoms. The majority of adults present with dysphagia and sore throat. Fever is absent in up to a third of patients and a voice change is present in over half. The diagnosis is often delayed in adults because most complain of a sore throat and dysphagia and do not have signs of airway obstruction. Epiglottitis should be suspect in those adult patients who complain of sore throat but have a normal oropharyngeal examination, muffled voice, or drooling. Finally, adults differ from children in that the inflammation is not confined to the epiglottis (as in children) but can also affect other structures such as the pharynx, uvula, base of the tongue, aryepiglottic folds, and false vocal cords.

121 *Staphylococcus aureus*.

122 B, C, and E. Epinephrine and dopamine, depending upon the dosage, either leave the pulmonary capillary wedge pressure unchanged or increase it, based on the amount of vasoconstriction. Dobutamine and isoproterenol hydrochloride increase cardiac output, decrease systemic vascular resistance, and decrease the pulmonary capillary wedge pressure. Amrinone hydrochloride is believed to cause vasodilation by increasing intracellular cAMP levels in smooth muscle. The action of amrinone hydrochloride is not related to sympathomimetic stimulation.

123–124: Questions

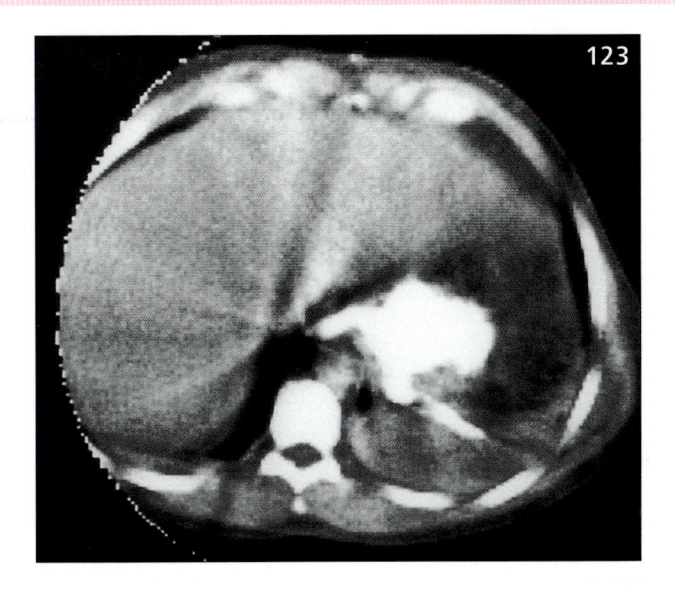

123 A 50-year-old male requires a splenectomy. He has placement of a closed suction drain for suspected pancreatic contusion. In the postoperative period, he develops fever and increased drainage. A CT scan is obtained (**123**). What is your diagnosis?

124 What are the class 4 antidysrhythmics?

125 A 70-kg (154-lb), 60-year-old female has a hysterectomy, bilateral salpingo-oophorectomy, omentectomy, and small bowel resection for ovarian carcinoma. She develops severe chest pain and shortness of breath 2 days postoperatively. She is admitted to the ICU with:

Temperature	37.8°C (100.0°F)	ABG	Room air
BP	130/90 mmHg (17.3/12.0 kPa)	PaO_2	55 mmHg (7.3 kPa)
Pulse	100/min	SaO_2	88%
RR	25/min	PCO_2	33 mmHg (4.4 kPa)
Tidal volume	720 ml	pH	7.36
Minute ventilation	18 l		

What is the diagnosis?

123–125: Answers

Secretion	Na+	K+	Cl-	HCO₃-
Stomach	30–90	4–12	50–150	70–90
Pancreatic	135–155	4–6	60–110	70–90
Jejunal	70–125	3.5–6.5	70–125	10–20

123 An increase in drainage in this patient is related to either a pancreatic fistula or a leak from the stomach. The drainage fluid can be analyzed for electrolyte content and amylase. This may help identify which is responsible for the drainage. The laboratory results above are in mmol/l (mEq/l). The CT scan identifies the stomach with a fistula with stomach contents directed toward the drain. A subphrenic collection is present. Alternative methods for identification of this problem may be to inject charcoal in the nasogastric tube and watch for charcoal coming from the drain. This charcoal test will not localize the level of the fistula. It could be either the stomach or small bowel. Gastric fistulas are a potential complication of splenectomy occurring at the level of the ligatures of the short gastric vessels. For this reason, many surgeons will oversew the area of the short gastric vessels which prevents gastric fistula formation.

124 Class 4 agents are the calcium antagonists, which prolong A–V nodal conduction and phase 2 of the action potential. Side effects include heart block, hypotension, and negative inotropic effects. These can be prevented by concomitant administration of small amounts of calcium. They can be used for chronic treatment of supraventricular tachyarrhythmias, as well as some of the hypertrophic cardiomyopathies.

125 This problem represents acute deadspace disease with hypoxemia. The minute ventilation is elevated and tidal volume is normal. Based on the formula for minute ventilation, deadspace ventilation must be increased.

Any increase in deadspace ventilation requires an increase in minute ventilation to maintain the same alveolar ventilation. There can be an increase in anatomic deadspace or an increase in alveolar deadspace. Anatomic deadspace (physiologic deadspace) is normally constant being 2.2 ml/kg of normal body weight. The pathologic causes for increased anatomic deadspace are increased work of breathing or CNS malfunction. Alveolar deadspace diseases are where ventilation is increased, but there is a decrease in pulmonary perfusion. This includes acute pulmonary embolus, acutely decreased cardiac output, acute pulmonary hypertension, alveolar septal destruction as in emphysema, and positive pressure ventilation with PEEP. There is a disparity between the minute ventilation and the $PaCO_2$. There is no evidence of shallow ventilation, so this is not compatible with increased anatomic deadspace. Further, the perfusion seems to be intact based upon the patient's vital signs. There is no evidence of hypermetabolism. Based on the blood gas analysis and patient's clinical history, she should be presumed to have a pulmonary embolus.

126–129: Questions

126 Which variable is associated with adequate treatment of acute asthma in a normal adult?
A Peak expiratory flow rate >200 l/min.
B Peak expiratory flow rate ≥300 l/min.
C Forced expiratory volume 1 <0.7 l.
D Forced expiratory volume 1 <1.5 l.
E Peak expiratory flow rate >100 l/min.

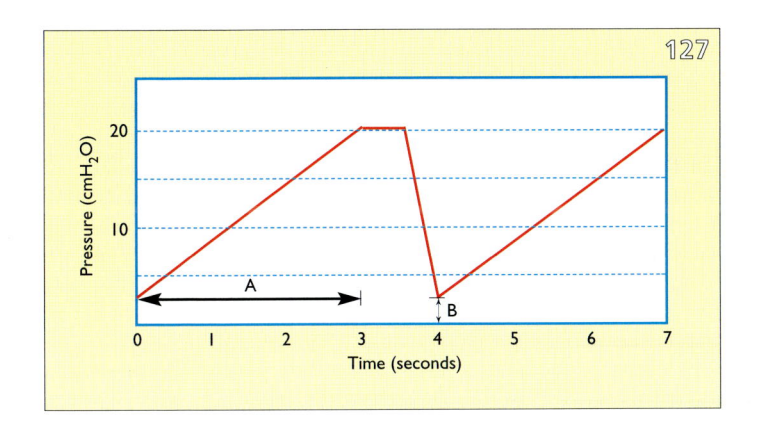

127 i. What mode of ventilation does this pressure time curve illustrate?
ii. When would it be most appropriately used?
iii. Why is the inspiration time period so long (demonstrated by arrow A), and what does arrow B indicate?

128 A 40-year-old female attended the hospital following an episode of chest pain. She is at 31 weeks gestation in her third pregnancy. Three weeks earlier she had been injured in a road traffic accident and required internal fixation of a right trimalleolar fracture. Clinical examination was unremarkable apart from a below-knee cast. She was discharged from the emergency room with simple analgesics. Two hours later she was readmitted having collapsed. Paramedics initiated CPR.
i. How does CPR differ in advanced pregnancy from the nonpregnant situation?
ii. What is the diagnosis?

129 What is the management of malignant hyperpyrexia?

126–129: Answers

126 B.

127 i. Pressure controlled ventilation with a reverse I:E ratio. This mode of ventilation is useful under circumstances of decreased lung compliance where a high airway pressure, and consequent risk of barotrauma, is to be avoided if at all possible.
ii. Higher airway pressures were thought to be helpful in recruiting alveoli that were atalectatic. Often PEEP was added to aid alveolar recruitment. Although application of PEEP invariably led to an increase in oxygenation, this was at the cost of lung damage (barotrauma) and increased mortality from complications such as pneumothorax. Ways were sought to reduce the effects of ventilation in noncompliant lungs.
iii. By increasing the time available for gas exchange in inspiration (arrow A), it may be possible to open previously closed alveoli that would otherwise not open except when subjected to a long period of positive pressure. The concept of reversing the normal inspiratory to expiratory ratio from 1:2 to 3:1 or 4:1 allows extra time for such alveoli to open. The effect of this is to reduce the time available for expiration. This may not be detrimental, as airway pressure does not return to zero before the next breath is applied. This has the effect of applying a PEEP to the patient's lungs that is known as 'auto PEEP' and is indicated by arrow B. Auto PEEP is applied by virtue of the way that the patient's lungs are being ventilated rather than by the application of a positive pressure through the ventilator circuitry. It is therefore believed to be more physiological.

128 i. It is necessary to maintain a left lateral tilt of at least 15° to avoid aortocaval compression by the gravid uterus. Delivering the baby may make the resuscitative attempts easier. If CPR has just been commenced then the baby may survive and skilled neonatal resuscitators and equipment are needed.
ii. Pulmonary thromboembolism.

129 The pathophysiology of this condition remains unclear. The basic cellular abnormality during an attack is a rise in the intracellular calcium concentration. This causes an increased ATP consumption and uncouples oxidative phosphorilation resulting in a hypermetabolic state. The first signs are tachycardia and a raised end tidal CO_2 followed by an increase in core temperature ≥2°C/hr (≥3.6°F/hr). The condition is inherited (chromosome 19). Known triggers include succinylcholine, volatile anesthetic agents, amide local anesthetics, caffeine, and phenothiazines.

The plan of management should be: (1) Remove any triggering agents (in the case of general anesthesia stop surgery as soon as is possible). (2) Hyperventilate the patient's lungs with 100% oxygen. (3) Prepare dantrolene and administer immediately – initially 2.5 mg/kg, with 1 mg/kg repeated every 10–15 minutes titrated to clinical response. The maximum does is 10 mg/kg. (4) Institute appropriate monitoring. This includes capnography, invasive arterial pressure monitoring, and a urinary catheter. (5) Measure serum urea, electrolytes, and glucose concentrations. Perform ABG analysis. (6) Correct hyperkalemia and acidosis. (7) Institute active cooling of the patient, topically to the skin, intravenously, and peritoneally. Cardiopulmonary bypass and ECMO have also been used. (8) Give mannitol and frusemide to promote diuresis.

130–132: Questions

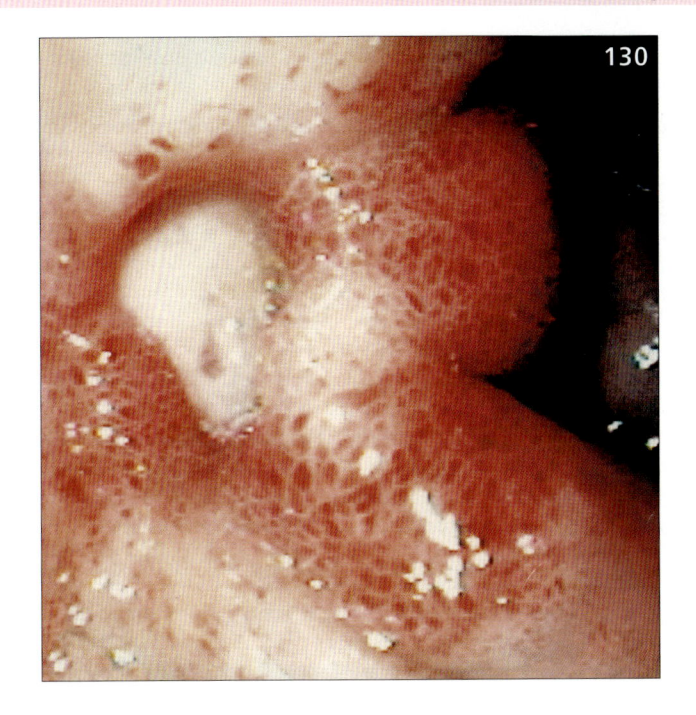

130 A patient presents to the hospital with a bleeding duodenal ulcer (130). The patient had an uncomplicated clinical course.
i. What are conditions associated with duodenal ulcers?
ii. Which additional tests should be performed?
iii. What is the appropriate therapy in the outpatient setting?

131 Describe the appropriate diagnostic work-up and differential diagnosis of effusions.

132 A 61-year-old male is resuscitated from a cardiac arrest 3 days after pancreatoduodenectomy. Twenty-four hours after the arrest the patient has a HR of 100/min, a BP of 118/76 mmHg (15.7/10.1 kPa), and good urine output. Neurologic examination reveals pupils with light reflexes, no spontaneous or roving eye on movements, and absent on motor reflexes. Discuss the neurologic prognosis for this patient.

130–132: Answers

130 i. *Helicobacter pylori* has been shown to be the causative agent in patients with chronic active gastritis and has been strongly linked to peptic ulcer disease, in the absence of other factors such as NSAIDs or the Zollinger–Ellison syndrome. This bacterium has been found in more than 95% of duodenal ulcers and 80% of gastric ulcers.

ii. A number of highly sensitive and specific tests are available to diagnose the presence of *H. pylori*, including serology for immunoglobulin G antibodies, breath tests of urease activity using orally administered ^{14}C- or ^{13}C-labeled urea, and endoscopically obtained histologic specimen and rapid urease tests. A fasting gastrin level should be obtained in patients with therapy resistant or multiple ulcers, complicated disease, or associated diarrhea, hypercalcemia, and prominent gastric folds.

iii. Generally a 6–8 week course of antisecretory therapy using an H_2-receptor antagonist or a proton-pump inhibitor has been used to treat duodenal ulcers. Whenever *H. pylori* infection is present, antibiotic treatment is indicated using a variety of effective drug regimens. This has been shown to result in a low ulcer recurrence. The long-term strategy after a hemorrhage remains under debate, but eradication therapy needs to be added to maintenance antisecretory treatment and surgery.

131 Effusion can be classified as either transudate or exudate. An effusion is deemed exudative if pleural fluid protein/serum protein ratio is >0.5, or pleural fluid lactate dehydrogenase (LDH)/serum LDH is >0.6, or pleural fluid LDH >2/3 upper normal limit for serum. Other commonly used tests include total fluid protein of more than 39 g/l (3.9 g/dl) and a specific gravity >1.016. If none of these criteria are met then the effusion is a transudate and the underlying medical disease is treated. Drainage is only needed if respiratory dysfunction occurs. If the effusion is exudative, additional studies such as cytology, amylase, complete blood count, bacterial cultures, and pH are obtained. Surgery is more commonly indicated. The presence of bacteria defines empyema.

132 This patient suffered global cerebral hypoxemia-ischemia injury following cardiac arrest. Primary respiratory failure, profound hypertension, and anesthetic problems can also lead to global ischemia. The best neurologic recovery is seen in patients who have a short duration of coma. Patients who remain in coma at 7–14 days after global ischemic infarct to the brain are unlikely to ever become independent. Patients who are comatose 1 month later are unlikely to regain consciousness. Individual neurologic signs suggesting recovery after global hypoxemic-ischemic eye insults are related to certain brain stem reflexes at the time of the initial examination. Absent light reflexes during the initial eye examination place the patient in a very poor prognostic category. The presence of a pupillary light reflex with the return of spontaneous eye opening and conjugant eye movements accompanied by motor response, improves the prognosis for regaining independence. Based upon this patient's examination at 24 hours, independent function is very unlikely.

133–136: Questions

133 A 37-year-old female is undergoing resection of a renal carcinoma that extends into the renal vein and the inferior vena cava. She is being monitored with an arterial line, pulmonary artery catheter, pulse oximeter, and capnograph under general anesthesia and has maintained stable cardiopulmonary parameters.

The inferior vena cava is cross-clamped and, immediately, the following changes are seen:

	Precross-clamp	Postcross-clamp
Systemic BP (mmHg (kPa))	114/65 (15.2/8.7)	108/60 (14.4/8.0)
Pulmonary artery pressure (mmHg (kPa))	21/12 (2.8/1.6)	47/29 (6.3/3.9)
Cardiac output (l/min)	5.2	4/9
Pulse oximetry (%)	99	96
End-tidal CO_2 (mmHg (kPa))	37 (4.9)	22 (2.9)

What is the most likely diagnosis?
A Accidental hyperventilation.
B Sudden hypovolemia.
C Pulmonary embolism.
D Ventilator disconnection.

134 This is the abdominal radiograph (**134a**) of a patient who underwent a diagnostic paracentesis for ascites fluid aspiration. What abnormality is seen on this radiograph?

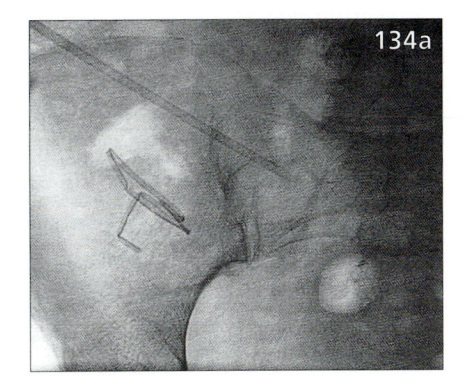

134a

135 Which organism is a common cause of pneumonia and urinary tract infections? It is facultative, Gram-negative, and has nonmotile rods with a large polysaccharide capsule. Culture reveals mucoid colonies that are lactose-fermenting on MacConkey's agar.

136 What are potential negative factors to consider when instituting pressure controlled ventilation with a reverse I:E ratio?

133–136: Answers

133 C. Capnography is an invaluable monitor of both pulmonary and myocardial performance in the operating room and ICU. Alterations in end-tidal CO_2 may be caused by equipment malfunction, changes in alveolar ventilation, or alterations in delivery of CO_2 to the lungs. Sudden decreases in end-tidal CO_2 are associated with sudden hyperventilation, ET obstruction, or disconnection from mechanical ventilation. It may also occur from a sudden decrease in cardiac output, resulting from myocardial dysfunction or hypovolemia. Pulmonary embolism of clot, air, fat, or amniotic fluid may also cause a rapid reduction in end-tidal CO_2 levels. In this patient, the abrupt decrease in end-tidal CO_2 coupled with the development of pulmonary hypertension while maintaining systemic hemodynamics, is most likely to have been caused by embolization of the tumor to the pulmonary circulation. Pulmonary hypertension would not be expected to result from any of the other choices.

134 The radiograph shows a retained portion of the paracentesis catheter. The catheter sheered off as it was removed from the abdomen. This is a technical error that can be avoided by careful attention to technique. Catheter-through-the-needle devices should be avoided. Catheter-over-the-needle devices or a Seldinger technique are preferred. Removal of this catheter was accomplished in this case under fluoroscopy with a wire loop (**134b**).

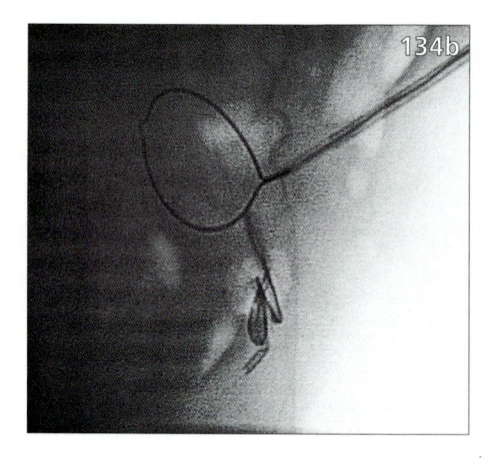

135 *Klebsiella pneumoniae*.

136 (1) Only pressure and time are set for ventilation therefore it is possible that an inadequate tidal volume may result. This is especially the case if the reverse I:E is so enthusiastically applied that insufficient time for expiration is allowed. The auto PEEP increases to such a degree that the patient becomes unventilated. Tidal and minute volume must always be closely monitored for this type of ventilation. (2) The mean intrathoracic pressure may be still be quite high utilizing this mode of ventilation, thus barotrauma can still occur. (3) Patients do not tolerate this mode of ventilation very easily. It feels uncomfortable to breathe with an abnormally long inspiratory phase and then be given insufficient time to exhale. For the reason heavy sedation and possibly paralysis is indicated, which may lead to artificial depression of blood pressure and consequent inadequate perfusion pressures. Sedation should be at the minimum level to allow tolerance of an inverse ratio ventilatory mode.

137, 138: Questions

137 A patient with multiple lower extremity fractures is admitted to the ICU. The urine is as shown (**137**). How would you diagnose and treat this problem?

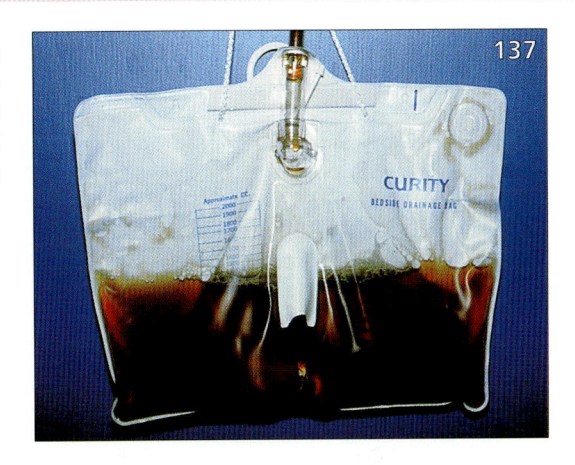

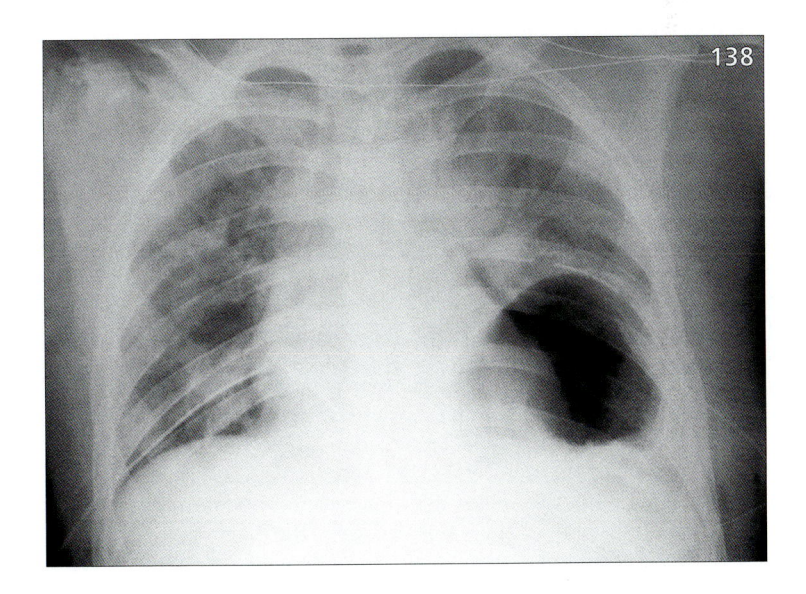

138 A 32-year-old emergency room physician was stabbed in the left chest by a psychotic patient. The stabwound is in the area of the sixth intercostal space in the anterior axillary line (**138**). The patient appears clinically stable. The next step in the management is:
A Diagnostic peritoneal lavage.
B Thoracoscopy.
C Laparoscopy.
D Laparotomy.
E Observation.
F Upper gastrointestinal study.

137, 138: Answers

137 The causes of myoglobinuria include compartment syndrome, the fairly uncommon thigh compartment syndrome, and massive soft-tissue injuries. Initial diagnosis of myoglobinuria can be obtained by a urine dipstick. If the dipstick is positive for blood, but the urinalysis is negative for RBCs, this implies myoglobinuria. If there is evidence of compartment syndrome, a fasciotomy is needed. Elevation of creatine phosphokinase levels with significant muscular injury can be used to confirm and monitor treatment. Treatment specific for myoglobinuria is largely supportive with high volume resuscitation accompanied by diuretic therapy. The purpose is to prevent myoglobin precipitation and renal injury. Additional therapy can include the use of mannitol which acts both as a diuretic and as an oxygen radical scavenger, further diminishing the renal injury. In elderly patients with cardiac disease, this high volume therapy must be carefully monitored. A urine output of more than 100 ml/hr is optimal and indeed up to a liter has been described as being beneficial. As the urine becomes clearer and the creatine phosphokinase reduced towards normal, the volume resuscitation can be decreased and finally stopped. Sodium bicarbonate has been prescribed historically as a form of alkalinization of the urine, but probably has minimal role. Its benefit is really only seen in those patients who have a massive diuresis.

138 C. Injury to the diaphragm occurs in 10% of penetrating chest traumas, but the diagnosis is made preoperatively in as few as 30% of patients. Complications include herniation of abdominal structures, bleeding, hemothorax, and missed visceral injuries. The injuries may be unrecognized because the defects are often very small, but enlarge over the ensuing years. Herniation with visceral incarceration usually occurs within 2 years of the injury and can present with pleural sepsis or bowel obstruction. The work-up of a stable patient who has only a pneumothorax can include thoracoscopy or laparoscopy. Thoracoscopy is efficient and can be performed via a pre-existing tube thoracostomy site. If, as in this case, there is a gross abnormality to the diaphragm or there are peritoneal findings, laparotomy is mandated to repair the probable intra-abdominal injuries. As a general rule, a gunshot wound is associated with up to 95% rate of severe abdominal trauma requiring surgery whereas stab wounds may require surgery in only one-third of patients. Trauma anterior to the anterior axillary lines is associated with an incidence of visceral injury approaching 70% whereas flank injuries are associated with a 30% rate. Flank and posterior injuries, however, may result in a colon injury that is missed until late sepsis develops. The diaphragm should be repaired with radially placed interrupted nonabsorbable sutures. In patients who are found to have gross contamination from visceral perforation, the affected hemithorax should be irrigated following control of the visceral leak. Some centers note a high incidence of positive *Candida* cultures in patients with gastric perforations.

139, 140: Questions

139 A 57-year-old male was admitted to ICU 10 days ago for pseudomonas pneumonia, necessitating continued ventilatory support for the past 7 days. The patient had a low grade temperature and right upper quadrant pain on palpation. The ultrasound and CT scan (**139a, b**), and laboratory findings are shown.
i. What is the diagnosis?
ii. What should be the course of therapy?

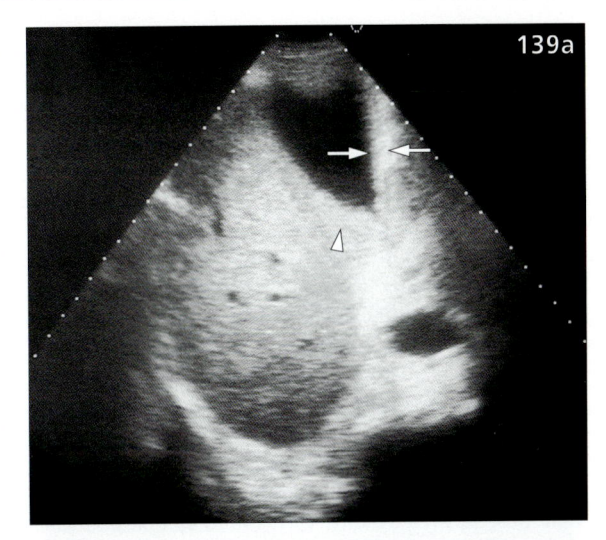

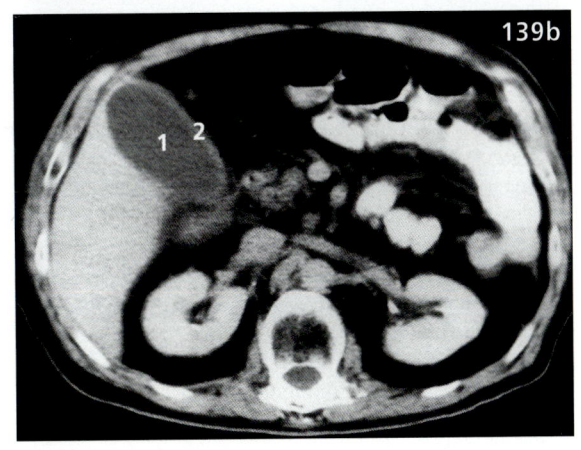

WBC 18 x 10⁹/l (18,000/mm³)
Bilirubin 60 µmol/l (3.5 mg/dl)
Alkaline phosphatase 124 u/l
Alanine transaminase 51 u/l

140 i. Define ARDS.
ii. What strategies of ventilation are recommended when ventilating a patient with ARDS?

139, 140: Answers

139 i. This patient has acute acalculous cholecystitis. The ultrasound scan (**139a**) shows that there is biliary sludge (arrowhead) in the gallbladder and a thickened gallbladder wall (arrows). The CT scan (**139b**) shows a distended gallbladder (1) filled with sludge with a thickened gallbladder wall (2).

ii. Acute acalculous cholecystitis is inflammation of the gallbladder in the absence of calculi. It occurs in patients with chronic debilitating disease and superimposed critical illness, trauma, or major burn injury. It is associated with decreased gastrointestinal motility and prolonged ileus. Risk factors include mechanical ventilation, hyperalimentation, dehydration and fasting, narcotics, massive blood transfusions, open wounds, abscesses, and chronic renal failure. A male predominance of up to 7 to 1 exists and the average age of symptoms is around 60 years old. About 2–15% of all acute cholecystitis is acalculous in nature. In trauma patients, acute acalculous cholecystitis may occur 1 week to 1 month after the initial trauma. Diagnostic use of a nuclear scan can be performed in the ICU with a 100% sensitivity and 90% specificity for acute acalculous cholecystitis. However, there can be false-negative nuclear scans. Cholescintigraphy using the synthetic octapeptide of cholecystokinin, sincalide, may yield false positive results. Ultrasound can be performed at the bedside and is positive if the gallbladder wall is 4 mm (0.2 in) or greater, there is pericholecystic fluid, subserosal edema in the absence of ascites, intramural gas, or sloughing of the mucosal membrane. The presence of biliary sludge is a minor criterion used for diagnosis. There have been reports that patients have been conservatively observed successfully and unsuccessfully. Due to the lack of correlation between symptomatology and pathology and a high incidence (59%) of necrosis and gangrene on pathologic review, cholecystectomy is the definitive procedure of choice. The mortality rate in these patients remains unacceptably high and early suspicion is warranted with therapy.

140 i. ARDS is associated with a generalized systemic inflammatory response syndrome and is defined as an acute onset, noncardiogenic pulmonary edema resulting from an increase in lung permeability leading to intractable hypoxemia and bilateral diffuse infiltrates on chest X-ray. Hypoxemia is defined as a PaO_2/FiO_2 ratio of <200 mmHg (26.3 kPa) regardless of the level of PEEP. A wedge (pulmonary artery occlusion) pressure of <18 mmHg (2.4 kPa) defines noncardiogenic pulmonary edema.

ii. Ventilation is very difficult due to the poor compliance that results from the protein leak into the lungs. The clinician should be familiar with the ventilator they are using and the mode of ventilation used to facilitate ventilation. Application of PEEP usually improves oxygenation but increases the likelihood of barotrauma, therefore a ventilating plateau pressure of no greater than 35 cmH$_2$O should be tolerated. Tidal volumes should be decreased down to 5 ml/kg if necessary. An acceptable SaO_2 should be >90%, and due to the necessity of keeping airway pressures minimal $PaCO_2$ should be permitted to rise unless contraindications (e.g. head injury) exist. FiO$_2$ should also be minimized where possible, but this may be difficult to achieve in the light of the reduced ventilation pressures. Where oxygenation continues to be inadequate, sedation, paralysis, and position changes (prone ventilation) are possible therapeutic maneuvers.

141–144: Questions

141 Methods of increasing mean airway pressure include all of the following except:
A Increased tidal volume.
B Decreased respiratory rate.
C Decreased inspiratory flow.
D Addition of end-inspiratory pause.
E Addition of PEEP.

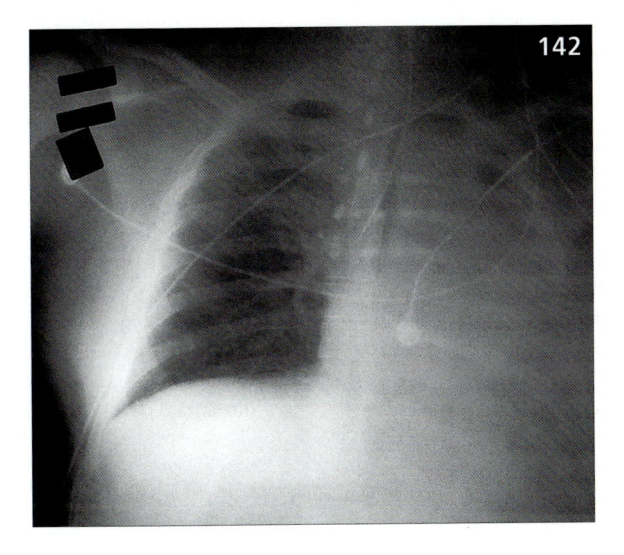

142 This chest radiograph (**142**) was obtained on a patient with decreased breath sounds. What is your diagnosis?

143 What are the class 3 antidysrhythmics?

144 A 72-year-old cachectic-appearing female presents to the emergency room with complaints of difficulty swallowing for 6 months with a recent worsening in severity. The patient complains of new onset of nausea and vomiting with a weight loss of 18 kg (40 lb) over 6 months. A work-up is in progress to evaluate an esophageal mass.

Height 1.65 m (5 ft 5 in)
Weight 45 kg (99 lb)
Total protein 50 g/l (5.0 g/dl)
Albumin 30 g/l (3.0 g/dl)

i. Define the three types of malnutrition. Which does this patient exhibit?
ii. Identify and explain which type of malnutrition places a patient at greatest risk for refeeding complications.
iii. What is the body's adaptive mechanism for starvation?
iv. List the three fuels used by the human body and which is the major storage fuel.

141–144: Answers

141 B. Mean airway pressure is measured as the area under the pressure–time curve during both inspiration and expiration, divided by the time of a total respiratory cycle. It is affected by peak airway pressure, duration of positive pressure ventilation, PEEP, inspiratory flow, RR, and flow waveform as well as respiratory system compliance and resistance. Increasing mean airway pressure is an effective way to improve oxygenation if alveolar recruitment is possible. Otherwise, alternative ventilator adjustments and patient treatment modalities may be necessary to improve arterial oxygenation.

142 The differential diagnosis of a chest radiograph which shows a whited-out lung is pleural effusion versus total lung collapse. This chest radiograph illustrates total lung collapse because of the tracheal and mediastinal shift toward the side of the whited-out area of the lung. Massive pleural effusion with mediastinal shift occurs away from the lesion because of the space occupying potential of the pleural fluid. The chest film also identifies the cause of the lung collapse as a right main stem bronchus intubation. This occurs on intubation or with ET tube movement during ICU care. With flexion and extension of the neck, the ET tube can move 4–6 cm (1.6–2.4 in).

143 Class 3 agents include bretylium and amiodarone. These agents prolong all the phases of the action potential. Bretylium blocks norepinephrine (noradrenaline) release and can cause hypotension. It is used to treat refractory ventricular arrhythmias. Amiodarone has less proarrhythmic effects and acts against supraventricular dysrhythmias as well as ventricular ones, with minimal direct cardiac depression. However, it has an extremely long half-life, and is associated with significant vasodilation, which can persist for days to weeks. This can be particularly problematic following a cardiac transplant and may require maintenance with an alpha-agonist agent for some days. Side effects include pulmonary fibrosis, hepatic dysfunction, bradycardia, and occasional proarrhythmic effects.

144 i. Marasmus (this patient) is defined as a loss of skeletal muscle and body fat with preservations of visceral proteins. Kwashiorkor is defined as a loss of visceral protein with preservation of body muscle and fat. Marasmus-Kwashiorkor is described as a combination of the two clinical states.
ii. Marasmus malnutrition places a patient at greatest risk for refeeding complications. Stress or injury mediated by hormonal and cytokine responses causes an increase in protein loss from both skeletal muscle and viscera that leads to hypoalbuminemia and anergy, causing an adult Kwashiorkor-like syndrome.
iii. The body adapts to starvation or insufficient exogenous energy supply by reducing energy expenditure and by a decrease in the basal metabolic rate, thereby reducing the rate of deterioration of body triglycerides.
iv. The three fuels used by the human body are carbohydrates, proteins, and lipids. Lipids or triglycerides are the major storage fuels of the body.

145, 146: Questions

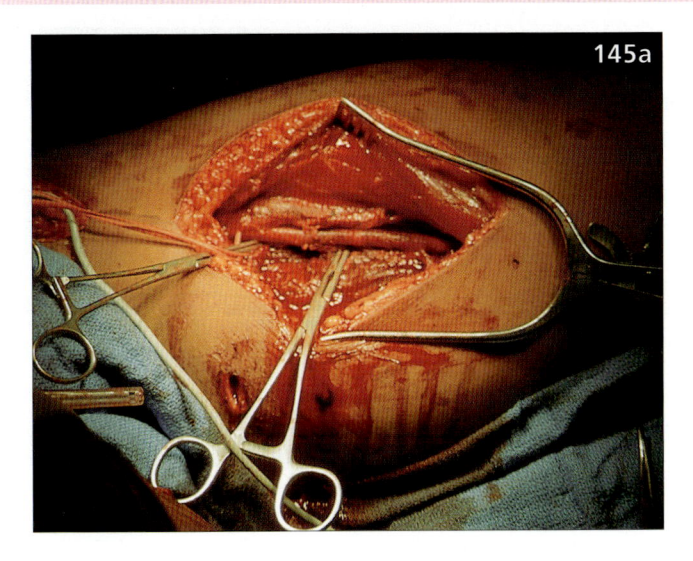

145 This patient suffered a gunshot to the thigh that transected the superficial femoral vein and contused the superficial femoral artery (**145a**). What are the options for reconstruction?

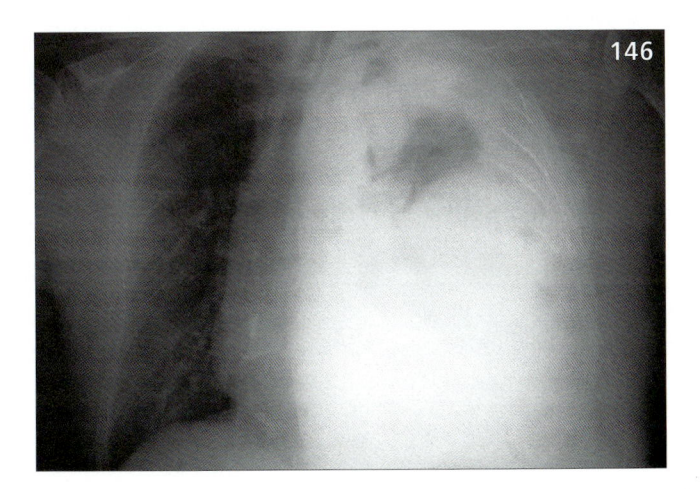

146 This patient is admitted to your ICU after a motor vehicle accident where he has sustained rib fractures. He is complaining of shortness of breath and has distended neck veins on examination. He has hypotension. The chest radiograph is obtained (**146**). What is your diagnosis and treatment?

145, 146: Answers

145 The contused segment of artery needs to be resected. The vein should be ligated. If the remnant of the venous system is intact, the likelihood of developing significant venous stasis is remote, but should be considered. This can be evaluated intraoperatively by duplex studies of the saphenous vein. If there is evidence of excessive venous pressure due to lack of outflow, the vein might be reconstructible with a saphenous graft. Some centers have advocated in rare instances the use of Gortex grafts for venous reconstruction, but usually in relatively high flow sites, such as the common femoral or iliac veins when there are no other options. Options for the artery include ligation (although this may lead to long-term problems), primary repair (although the damage here is too extensive), or bypass. Ideally, bypass can be performed with a saphenous graft. However, in this case there is already a deep venous injury, requiring use of a vein harvested from the opposite leg. If there is no injury of that leg, this is an option. Another method is to use Gortex material (**145b**).

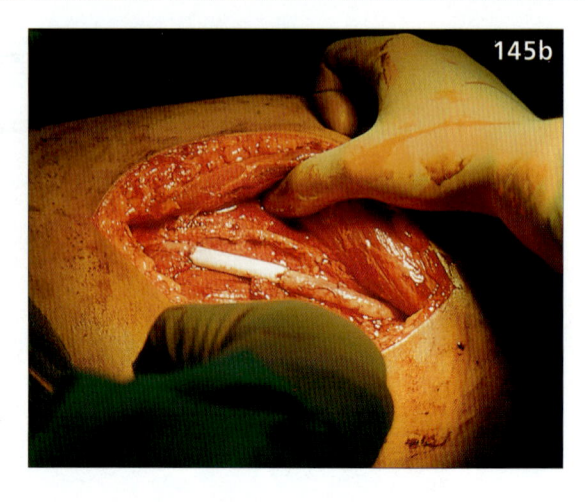

146 When this patient's symptoms are put together with the accompanying chest radiograph, the diagnosis is a massive hemothorax. Since the hemothorax is a space occupying lesion, it will cause shift of the mediastinum, heart, and tracheal structures away from the lung with hemothorax. Radiographically, this must be distinguished from a patient with total lung collapse where the shift is toward the side of the collapse. The treatment for hemothorax is placement of a chest tube. Massive blood loss through a chest tube may indicate the need for thoracotomy. Intercostal arterial bleeding and major lung laceration will cause massive blood loss. With pulmonary parenchymal laceration, the blood loss will stop as soon as the hemothorax is evacuated and the lung completely expanded.

147–149: Questions

147 A 67-year-old male with respiratory failure secondary to COPD is receiving mechanical ventilation. A chest radiograph taken on the second hospital day is shown (**147**). The patient is stable from a cardiorespiratory standpoint. Enteral nutrition is to be initiated as it is anticipated that the patient will require a prolonged period of ventilatory support. Which of the following would be most appropriate in the management of this patient?
A Initiation of enteral feeds with a high lipid and low carbohydrate content.
B Place the nasoenteric tube to low suction for 24 hours to assess gastric residuals.
C Placement of a thoracostomy tube.
D Withdraw the nasoenteric tube 10 cm (4 in) and begin enteral feeds with an elemental diet.

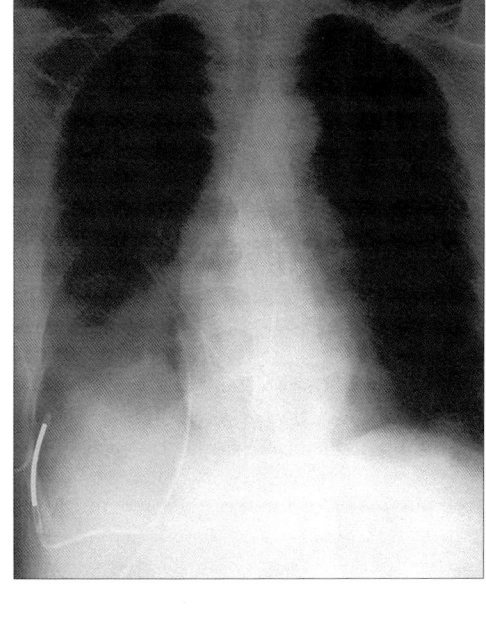

148 An 82-year-old female presents with exertional syncope. Her exercise tolerance has declined over the last 2 years, such that she now has dyspnea when climbing one flight of stairs. She has no cardiac risk factors. Echocardiography demonstrates a mean aortic valve gradient of 32 mmHg (4.3 kPa), a planimetrically determined valve area of 0.6 cm^2 (0.1 in^2) and severe reduction of left ventricular function with concentric hypertrophy. Discuss the echocardiographic result, further diagnostic tests, prognosis, and therapeutic options for this patient.

149 A 25-year-old male presents to emergency department with a gunshot wound to the epigastric area. There is no exit wound. On examination, his systolic BP is 90 mmHg (12.0 kPa), his HR is 110/min, and his RR 20/min. His breath sounds are equal bilaterally and he has distended neck veins. He is awake and alert with no movement of the lower extremities. Most likely, the etiology of his hypotension is:
A Hypovolemic shock.
B Air embolus.
C Tension pneumothorax.
D Pericardial tamponade.
E Neurogenic shock.

147–149: Answers

147 C. The nasoenteric tube has penetrated the lung, run along the diaphragm and turned upwards along the rib cage. As a result, the patient has developed a pneumothorax that requires immediate drainage. The nasoenteric tube should be removed and reinstated when the patient is in stable condition. A radiograph should then be taken to confirm the position of the tube in the stomach.

148 This woman has severe aortic stenosis. Echocardiography is very accurate at identifying this if several types of determination are employed. Valve gradients may be determined by the continuity equation. A mean gradient over 50 mmHg (6.7 kPa) and a peak >60 mmHg (8.0 kPa) are very suggestive of severe stenosis. The aortic valve area may be determined by Doppler (i.e. velocity) or planimetry (i.e. direct visualization of the valve orifice) as well as aortic valve resistance (which is independent of gradient and flow). All these results correlate strongly with gradients and areas determined by cardiac catheterization using the Gorlin formula. Catheterization is usually requested to assess coronary anatomy. Reduced left ventricular function in this woman probably accounts for the relatively low measured gradient. Symptomatic medical treatment of severe aortic stenosis in the elderly results in a 2-year mortality rate of about 50%, about half of these from sudden death. Surgical treatment is associated with a mortality rate of about 3–5%, dependent on age, urgency, reoperation, left ventricular function, coronary artery disease, atrial fibrillation, and comorbidity. Survival following AVR is less than for the general population, being 75% at 5 years and 60% at 10 years – a distinct improvement over medical therapy. Percutaneous balloon aortic valvuloplasty has a high complication rate (25% with aortic regurgitation, cardiac rupture, stroke, myocardial infarction, or conduction abnormalities) and a high recurrence rate (50–75% in 9 months) with a 30% mortality in 1 year. Its best indication may be in those patients who are not operative candidates, in whom it may improve function temporarily so that an operation becomes possible.

149 D. The usual cause of hypotension after penetrating injury is hemorrhagic shock; however, this is inconsistent with this patient's distended neck veins. A large intravascular volume deficit occurs with hemorrhagic shock which should produce flat neck veins. Neurogenic shock is possible in this patient, however, this produces vasodilation which allows blood to pool in the extremities and is inconsistent of the physical finding of distended neck veins. The complex of hypotension and distended neck veins after trauma is classic for pericardial tamponade, tension pneumothorax, air embolization, and myocardial infarction or severe myocardial contusion. Air embolization is unlikely in a spontaneously breathing patient, but does occur when patients are subject to positive pressure ventilation. The finding of equal bilateral breath sounds is not consistent with the diagnosis of tension pneumothorax. A gunshot wound crossing or entering the mediastinum partnered with hypotension and distended neck veins is consistent with pericardial tamponade.

150–152: Questions

150 Total parenteral nutrition in very malnourished patients may be associated with with 'refeeding syndrome'.
i. Describe the major fuel sources affected by 'refeeding syndrome'.
ii. Which electrolytes are affected by 'refeeding syndrome'?
iii. Describe the effects of hypophosphatemia and 'refeeding syndrome'.
iv. Does enteral nutrition cause 'refeeding syndrome'?

151 A patient returns to the ICU after the performance of the tracheostomy in the operating room. After transfer to the ICU bed, the patient becomes agitated and experiences difficulty breathing. What would you do?

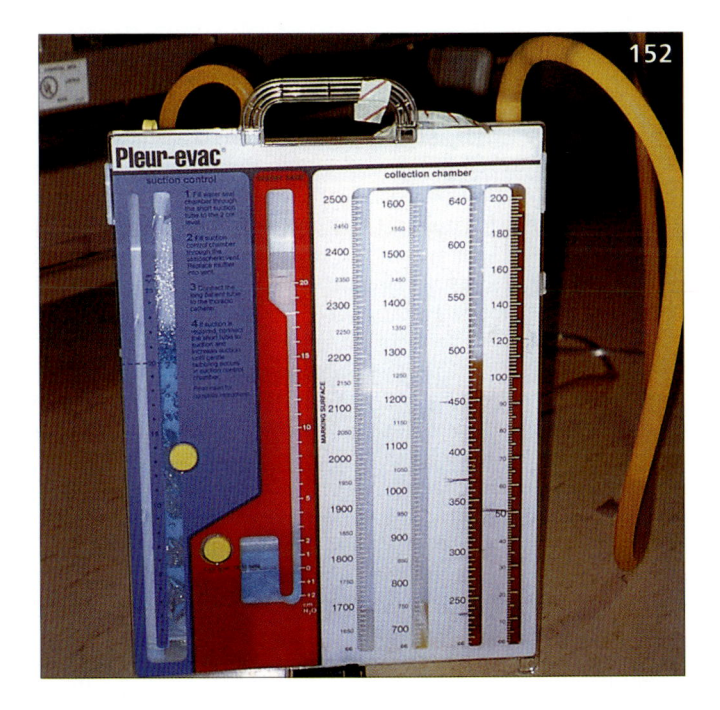

152 Modern thoracostomy drainage systems are patterned on the classic three bottle method. Explain the function of each of the columns in the device shown (**152**).

150–152: Answers

150 i. The fuel sources affected by refeeding syndrome are carbohydrates and lipids. The metabolic response to refeeding is a shift from body fat to carbohydrate as the major fuel source. Glycogenolysis and gluconeogenesis are reduced and fatty acid mobilization from adipose tissues is inhibited by insulin. Cellular uptake of glucose, potassium, phosphorus, and magnesium are all enhanced by the action of insulin.

ii. Refeeding syndrome has typically been thought of as severe hypophosphatemia which presents as one of the most serious metabolic complications of nutritional support. There is a movement of phosphorus from the extracellular to the intracellular space for the synthesis of phosphorylated compounds. Potassium and magnesium are also shifted intracellularly causing hypokalemia and hypomagnesemia.

iii. Hypophosphatemia may occur rapidly or may be delayed by several days in patients who have normal body stores of phosphorus. Severe hypophosphatemia (<0.32 mmol/l; <1.0 mg/dl) is associated with severe life-threatening complications that include respiratory failure, cardiac abnormalities, CNS dysfunction, RBC dysfunction, leukocyte dysfunction, and difficulty in weaning from the ventilator.

iv. Enteral feeding can cause refeeding syndrome, although most attention has been focused on the syndrome with regard to total parenteral nutrition.

151 There are two circumstances to consider. One is the occurrence of a pneumothorax with the tracheostomy. Careful examination of the chest should be performed. If there are decreased breath sounds on one side of the chest and a hyperpercussion note is present, this confirms the diagnosis of the pneumothorax. The patient should be immediately placed on 100% FiO_2 and the pneumothorax decompressed through a needle or a tube thoracostomy. If breath sounds are not heard on either side, dislodgement of the tube must be suspected and an attempt to suction out the tracheostomy tube should be performed. If this is not possible, the tracheostomy tube has become dislodged. This is an absolute surgical emergency. The tracheostomy tube should be removed, the patient should be bag masked and attempted oral tracheal intubation can be made or, alternatively, an attempt made at placing a small ET tube through the surgical site. This can be aided by previously placed stay sutures. Another alternative is to place a pediatric laryngoscope blade through the surgical site into the trachea and either a tracheostomy tube or a small ET tube placed under direct vision.

152 The left-most column (blue in the picture) is the suction chamber. Tubing from the suction generator is connected to the collection device at this location. The height of the water column in this chamber determines the magnitude of the negative pressure applied to the pleural space. In the example the pressure is –20 cmH_2O. The center or red column is the water seal chamber. This is the location where pleural pressure is allowed to equilibrate with the negative pressure of the suction or atmospheric pressure if the patient is on only water seal. Retained air in the hemithorax will cause elevated pleural pressure which decompresses in the water seal chamber. This air leak manifests as bubbling in this chamber. The third chamber (white in the picture) is the collection chamber which traps fluid drained from the patient.

153–155: Questions

153 This is effluent from a diagnostic peritoneal lavage (**153**).
i. What is a positive lavage?
ii. What is the role of diagnostic peritoneal lavage in the ICU?

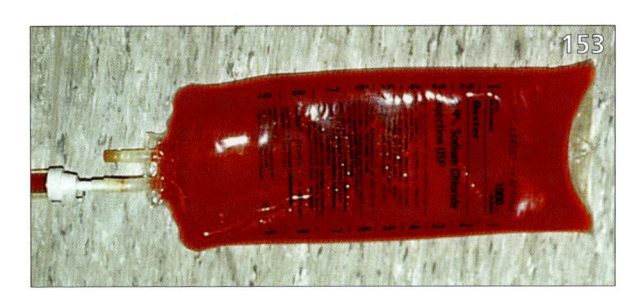

154 Are the following statements true or false?
A Patients with diaphragmatic paralysis are weaned in the supine position.
B Patients with lower cervical spine paralysis are weaned in the upright position.
C Mechanical ventilators trigger sensitivity and inspiratory flow rates determine the patient's work of breathing on the ventilator.
D Patients with chronic hypercapnia are best weaned with normal PCO_2.
E The work of breathing is increased when external PEEP exceeds auto PEEP.
F Lipid calories produce more CO_2 than carbohydrate calories.
G Hyperinflation impairs inspiratory muscle function.
H Increased dead space ventilation increases work of breathing.
I Increased work of breathing can be measured by determining the difference of the total O_2 consumption on mechanical ventilation and spontaneous breathing.
J The intrathoracic pressure effects of spontaneous breathing and positive pressure ventilation occur in the same direction.
K Normal inspiration decreases HR.
L Hyperinflation increases pulmonary vascular resistance.
M Low functional residual capacity increases pulmonary vascular resistance.
N Weaning patients increases venous return.
O Synchronous intermittent mandatory ventilation (SIMV), intermittent mandatory ventilation (IMV), and pressure support ventilation (PSV) weaning are more effective than spontaneous breathing trials.

155 A 24-year-old male who is noncompliant with his phenytoin presents to the emergency department with 10 seizures in the past 2 hours after being assaulted. What is the most important immediate action?
A Load with phenytoin 1,000 mg intravenous piggy-back (IVPB) over 20 minutes.
B Intramuscular injection of 1,500 mg of phosphenytoin.
C Administration of 2 mg of lorazepam.
D Secure the airway.
E Load with phenytoin 1,000 mg IVPB and obtain a CT of the patient's head.

153–155: Answers

153 i. A 'grossly positive' lavage has traditionally been taken as one that is so bloody that it is impossible to read printed material through it. In general, for blunt trauma, a positive diagnostic peritoneal lavage would include any of the following:
- 10 ml of gross blood on free aspiration.
- RBC $>1 \times 10^{11}$/l ($>100,000$/mm^3).
- WBC $>0.5 \times 10^{9}$/l (>500/mm^3).
- Bacteria on Gram stain.
- Food particles.
- Bile seen grossly.

The RBC count that is taken as an indication of positive lavage for penetrating trauma varies from institution to institution, with some taking as low as 1×10^{9}/l (1,000/mm^3) while others require 1×10^{10}/l (10,000/mm^3) depending on the rate of nontherapeutic laparotomies that each institution is willing to accept.

ii. Any trauma patient, or any patient at increased risk of intra-abdominal bleeding, who experiences sudden deterioration that can not be explained should be considered for diagnostic peritoneal lavage even if a previous one was 'normal'. Also, a diagnostic peritoneal lavage can be useful in assessing intra-abdominal sepsis, especially the possibility of an ischemic bowel.

154
A False.
B False.
C True.
D False.
E True.
F False.
G True.
H True.
I True.
J False.
K False.
L True.
M True.
N True.
O False.

155 D. Although all actions are important, the most important immediate step is to secure the airway.

156, 157: Questions

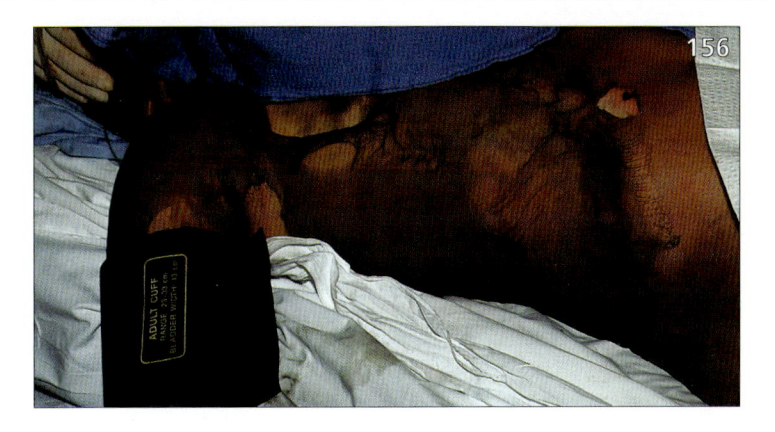

156 This 50-year-old farmer (**156**) suffered a 60% body surface area burn injury from an exploding gas tank. It was noted that there was increasing difficulty to ventilate the patient. Blood gases revealed a $PaCO_2$ of 50 mmHg (6.7 kPa), a PO_2 of 290 mmHg (38.7 kPa) and a pH of 7.30. The ventilator settings were a tidal volume of 700 ml, RR of 20/min, and FiO_2 of 100%. Peak inspiratory pressures have increased to 60 cm of water. The chest X-ray shows no interval change. He is paralyzed medically. The next step is:
A Pulmonary angiography.
B Reparalyze the patient.
C High frequency ventilation.
D Chest wall escharotomy.
E Bilateral chest tubes.

157 An elderly patient was admitted to the ICU because of worsening cardiac and respiratory failure. Shortly after this chest X-ray was obtained (**157**), she began to experience brisk hemoptysis. Discuss your management.

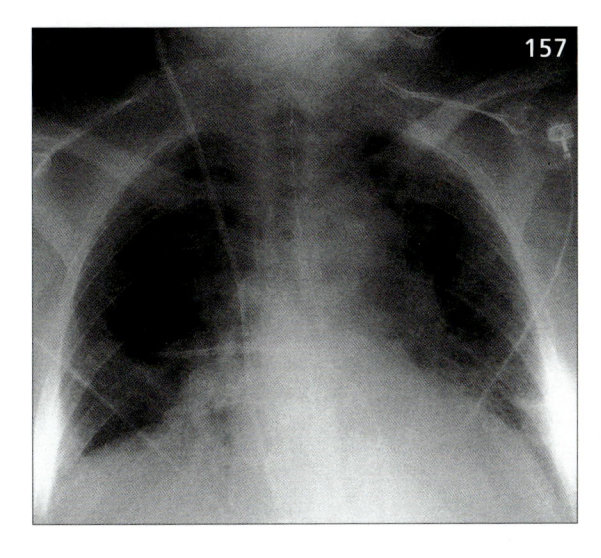

156, 157: Answers

156 D. Causes of increasing airway pressure on the ventilator include mechanical ones such as an obstructive or kinked ET tube, right main stem intubation, or bilateral/unilateral tension pneumothorax. Parenchymal causes include pulmonary edema, ARDS, or severe pneumonia. Pharmacologic causes include fentanyl rigidity. Burn patients who have a severe chest wall burn, as this patient has, may have a restrictive thoracic defect that requires bilateral escharotomy. The landmarks for this are from the axilla towards the anterior superior iliac spine or down to wherever the eschar ends. Inhalational burns can also be the cause of difficulty in oxygenating (and may be an additional problem in this case), although they usually are not associated acutely with severe restrictive defect and high airway pressures. Some centers have noted a decreased complication rate and an increased survival rate when using high frequency ventilation in this setting.

157 The chest X-ray demonstrates that the pulmonary artery occlusion catheter is too far advanced into the pulmonary artery, and thus may have resulted in pulmonary artery rupture. Risk factors for pulmonary artery occlusion catheter induced pulmonary arterial rupture include: pulmonary hypertension; hypothermia; over advancement; over inflation; coagulopathy; small body size. Initial management includes administering supplemental oxygen and keeping the patient upright. Should the blood loss appear so rapid as to threaten 'drowning' the opposite lung, the patient should be placed with the affected side down, but preferably still in reverse Trendelenburg. Simultaneous measures include withdrawing the catheter 1 cm (0.4 in) and trying to gently reinflate the balloon so as to occlude the vessel. If the bleeding is brief and stops, the catheter should be removed and the patient managed expectantly with serial chest X-rays (to rule out hemothorax), antibiotics, and correction of any coagulation abnormalities. If the bleeding continues, but is only intermittent and mild, one option is to perform angiographic embolization. The pulmonary artery occlusion catheter can be used for this purpose. If there is evidence of more severe bleeding the patient should be taken to the operating room. Induction should be performed with the patient in a relatively upright position, with the rigid bronchoscope immediately available. After induction, rigid bronchoscopy is used to suck out blood clots, obtain samples for culture, and to place a fogarty catheter to occlude the affected bronchus. The commonest site of bleeding is the right middle or lower lobes. The patient is left intubated with a single lumen tube that is large enough to allow flexible bronchoscopy and is continuously medically paralyzed. After 24 hours, under endoscopic observation, the bronchial balloon can be deflated. If there is no bleeding, after a further 24 hours the fogarty can be removed and the patient weaned from the ventilator.

158, 159: Questions

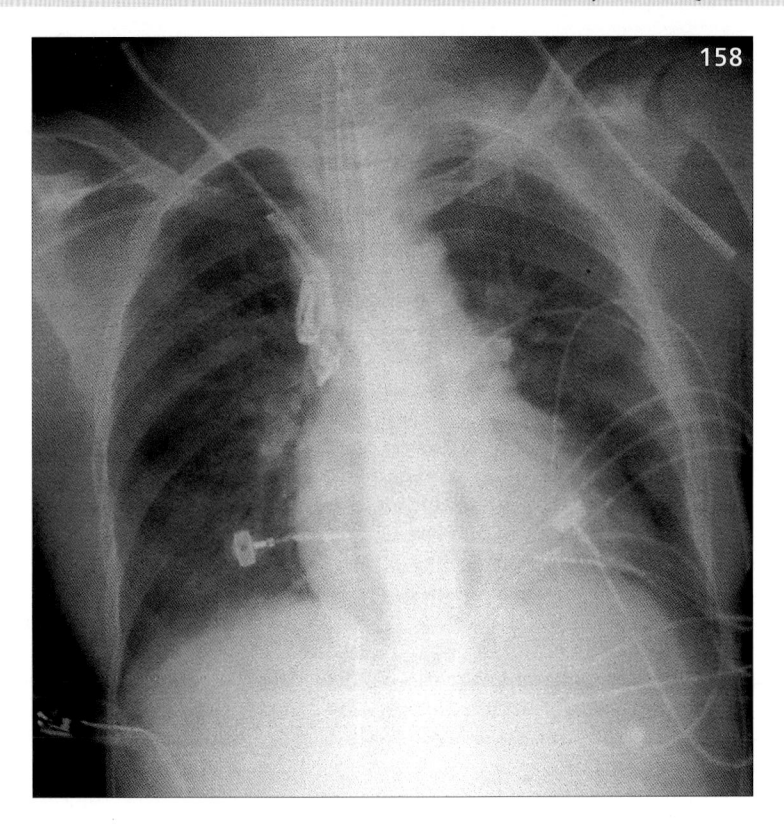

158 A 72-year-old male is admitted to the ICU following an emergency laparotomy for perforated colon. A decision is made to insert a pulmonary artery catheter to optimize hemodynamics. The pulmonary artery catheter can not be positioned with a good pulmonary artery trace. A chest X-ray is taken to determine the position of the catheter (158). Appropriate management might include all of the following except:
A Insert a guide wire through the pulmonary artery catheter under fluoroscopic guidance to aid in unknotting the catheter.
B Withdraw the catheter along with the introducer.
C Contact a surgeon to remove the catheter in an open fashion.
D Calibrate the transducers and determine cardiac output by thermodilution.

159 What are the relative merits of the use of crystalloid, colloid and/or hypertonic fluid resuscitation?

158, 159: Answers

158 D. Pulmonary artery catherization is associated with a number of complications. Dysrhythmias are common during insertion, and complete heart block may result in a patient with pre-existing left bundle branch block. Endobronchial hemorrhage can occur, as can pulmonary infarction. Tricuspid and pulmonary valvular damage may lead to endocarditis. Knotting of a pulmonary artery catheter usually occurs as a result of coiling of the catheter in the right ventricle. A number of techniques have been described to unknot the catheter, including attempts at withdrawal of the catheter and introducer, or insertion of a guidewire and manipulation of the catheter under fluoroscopy. Failing these techniques, or if the catheter is knotted around a cardiac structure such as the papillary muscles, surgical intervention may be required.

159 For years, this was an area of great debate. Briefly, the theoretical argument in favor of colloid solution was that the fluid 'stayed' in the intravascular space and it increased the intravascular colloid osmotic pressure, thereby further drawing fluid within the intravascular space and leading to further volume expansion. Arguments for crystalloid solution are a general intracellular as well as intravascular volume deficit exists which needs to be replaced, and in trauma and septic patients a diffuse capillary leak is prevalent so that colloid does not stay in the intravascular space anyway. To address the issue, several prospective, randomized studies have been done, with mixed results. Subsequently, a meta-analysis of these trials was done to help sort out the confusion. Essentially, there is a lower mortality rate with the use of crystalloid solution in trauma patients. Conversely, there seems to be a small, approximately 8%, mortality advantage with colloid solution in major elective surgery, such as abdominal aortic aneurysms. These differences may reflect the different physiologies of the trauma patient, who has had some measure of pre-existing shock, versus the elective surgical patient in whom preoperative and intraoperative shock did not exist.

Other solutions for volume expansion also exist. The most extensively studied is hypertonic saline. The theory is that infusion of a hypertonic solution will increase the tonicity of the intravascular space, thereby drawing intracellular water into the intravascular space. However, the results of clinical trials have been mixed for this as well. Although as a substitute for normotonic crystalloid solution for blunt trauma patients, hypertonic solutions appear acceptable, no clear advantage has been achieved over normotonic solutions. In addition, in burn patients, hypertonic solutions have led to an increased incidence of renal failure and death. Furthermore, hypertonic solutions have been associated with coagulopathies. Because of all this, hypertonic solutions have not become routine practice in the resuscitation of trauma victims.

160, 161: Questions

160 Briefly list the pulmonary manifestation of AIDS.

161 A 76-year-old female in the thoracic unit was doing well 2 days after a mitral valve replacement. She has been extubated. You are consulted because she has suddenly begun complaining of severe abdominal pain. On physical examination, she is awake and alert, but obviously in pain, sweating profusely. She says the pain is crampy and located mainly in the right upper quadrant. She has vomited 200 ml of bilious, guaiac positive fluid. She has a well healed lower midline scar from a hysterectomy 30 years ago. Her abdomen is nondistended and soft. Bowel sounds are active. You cannot elicit any specific point of increased tenderness on palpation.

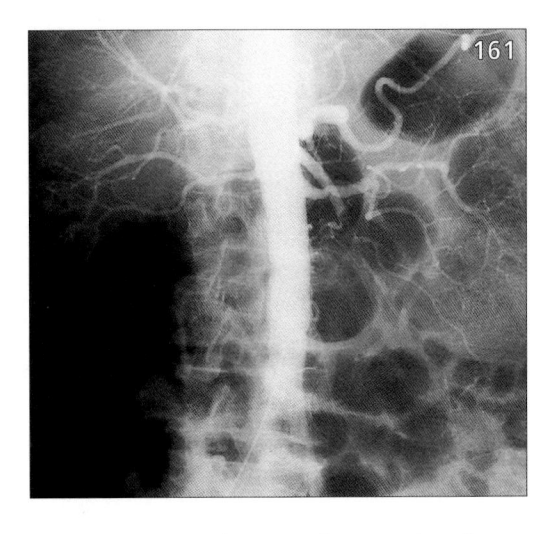

i. Your differential diagnosis is:
A Bowel obstruction.
B Mesenteric ischemia.
C Perforated viscus.
D Intra-abdominal infection.
E All the above.

ii. The first thing you obtain, after resuscitating the patient, does not include:
A Arteriogram.
B ECG.
C Flat plate of abdomen.
D Electrolytes, complete blood count, BUN, creatinine, and urine analysis.

iii. The abdominal X-ray is nonspecific. The electrolytes are normal, the WBC not elevated. Serum lactate is 3.5 mmol/l (mEq/l). Because the patient continues to show pain out of proportion to physical findings, an arteriogram is done (**161**), which shows an inverted meniscus sign 6 cm (2.4 in) from the origin of the superior mesenteric artery. With what diagnosis is this compatible?
A Acute mesenteric thrombosis.
B Chronic mesenteric ischemia.
C Acute mesenteric embolus.
D Mesenteric venous thrombosis.

iv. What steps should be avoided when attempting to optimize the patient for the operating room?
A Heparin infusion.
B Digitalis bolus.
C Oxygen.
D Pulmonary artery catheter.

160, 161: Answers

160 Opportunistic pneumonia including pneumocystitis with pneumonia, strongyloides, and toxoplasmosis. Pneumocystitis with pneumonia is the initial presentation in 50% of patients and 80% of AIDS patients have at least one episode. In patients who have been treated by aerosolized pentamidine, pneumothoraces are a risk because of necrosis of the lung concomitant with death of the organisms. In patients who have been treated with pentamidine, pneumocystitis with pneumonia presents basally, whereas in a patient who has not been treated with the pentamidine, the pneumocystitis with pneumonia presents more often in the upper lobes. Viral pneumonia (commonly cytomegalovirus). Pyogenic pneumonia. Mycobacterial pneumonia including 'atypical' strains such as *Mycobacterium avium intracellulare* and tuberculosis. Fungal disease. Pneumothorax related to pneumocystitis with pneumonia as mentioned above. Noninfectious complications including Kaposi's sarcoma, lymphoma (diffuse T-cell), and lymphocytic pneumonia. Nonpulmonary manifestations including lymphadenopathy.

161 i. E.
ii. A. You do not need an arteriogram until you have ruled out other causes of her abdominal pain. The abdominal X-ray will give you evidence of free air or bowel obstruction; laboratory results may show infection or other abnormalities. An ECG would rule out acute myocardial infarction or reveal new onset of atrial fibrillation.
iii. C. The history of acute onset of abdominal pain with a potential cardiac source would make one suspect an embolus to the mesenteric circulation (i.e. superior mesenteric artery). The inverted meniscus sign several centimeters from the origin of the superior mesenteric artery supports this diagnosis. Because of the large caliber of the vessel and its oblique take off from the aorta, emboli tend to favor the superior mesenteric artery. If there is no atherosclerotic narrowing of the origin of the artery, emboli tend to lodge at the level of the first major branch, the middle colic, sparing the first several jejunal branches, as well as the inferior pancreaticoduodenal. Acute mesenteric thrombosis tends to occlude the superior mesenteric artery at its origin, where atherosclerotic narrowing has already limited flow. Onset of abdominal pain tends to be insidious over several days. Chronic mesenteric ischemia can show occluded splanchnic arteries, but the diagnosis hinges on its association with the trial of postprandial abdominal pain, weight loss, and fear of eating. Mesenteric venous thrombosis tends to occur in younger patients with a hypercoagulable state. Symptoms are insidious in onset. The arteriogram is seldom diagnostic.
iv. B. Digitalis bolus has been shown to have vasoconstrictor effects on smooth muscle and must be avoided if possible. A heparin drip may stabilize a residual clot in the heart as well as prevent propagation of clot distal to the embolus in the superior mesenteric artery circulation. A pulmonary artery catheter may be required to optimize cardiac function and guide in fluid resuscitation.

162–164: Questions

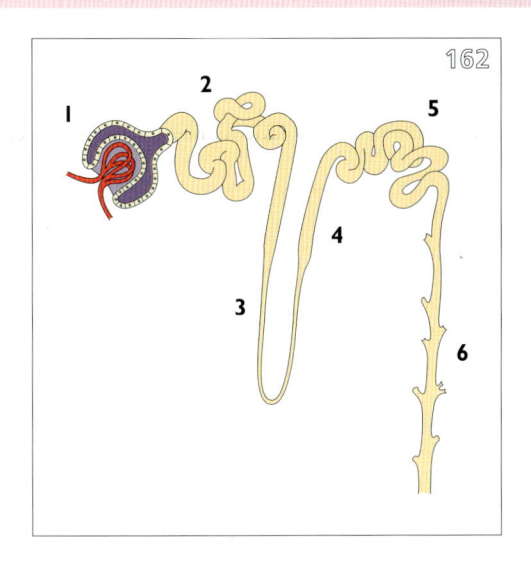

162 Match the diuretic to the portion of nephron with which it interacts (**162**).
A Spironolactone.
B Furosemide (frusemide).
C Mannitol.
D Thiazide diuretics.

163 With regard to ECMO which of the following statements are true?
A Veno-arterial bypass is preferable to veno–venous bypass when cardiac support is required.
B ECMO should not be instituted until a trial of conventional and unconventional ventilatory support has been tried for at least 48 hours.
C Repair of complex 'surgical' lesions may be done on or off ECMO (e.g. of congenital diaphragmatic hernia, laryngotracheal esophageal cleft).
D There is an absolute time limit of 72 hours on ECMO before irreversible complications ensue.
E A weight of 3 kg (6.6 lb) or greater is mandatory regarding vessel size for cannulation.

164 What does Ohm's law have to do with electrical injuries? In light of Ohm's law, which tissues are injured the worst with electrical current?

162–164: Answers

162 A and 6. Spironolactone is an example of a potassium sparing diuretic which acts at the level of the collecting duct tubule. Spironolactone competes with aldosterone for its receptor site, which decreases the excretion of K+ and H+ ions.

B and 4. Furosemide is a loop diuretic which inhibits the Na+, K+, and Cl− transport mechanism in the thick ascending loop of Henle. It reversibly binds to one of the Cl− binding sites on the tubular cell. The inhibition of Na+ transport decreases the interstitial hypertonicity in the medullary area which leads to a decrease in water reabsorption in the collecting tubule. Loop diuretics increase renal blood flow by approximately 40% and cause a redistribution of renal blood flow from the inner to the outer renal cortex.

C and 2. Mannitol, an osmotic diuretic, is freely filterable at the glomerulus, poorly reabsorbed and metabolically inert. Mannitol has little effect on Na+ reabsorption in the proximal tubule. Because mannitol is not reabsorbed, it primarily inhibits reabsorption of water. This water reabsorption results in a low tubular concentration of Na+ and, therefore, decreases the gradient for Na+ reabsorption. Additionally, mannitol increases renal blood flow to the medullary area, producing a partial washout effect of the medullary hypertonicity.

D and 5. Thiazide diuretics act at the distal convoluted tubule and also inhibit the sodium chloride transport system. The diuresis produced by thiazide diuretics is limited because this area of the nephron is only responsible for 5% of Na+ reabsorption.

163 A and C. With regard to time limits and ECMO there is no hard and fast rule for using conventional ventilatory support before instituting ECMO. A decision to begin ECMO is made on relatively strict criteria based on the alveolar arterial oxygen gradient, oxygenation index, and responses of the oxygenation and ventilation to conventional therapy, including nitric oxide. There are relative and absolute contraindications, such as severe intracranial hemorrhage, birth weight under 2 kg (4.4 lb), and severe congenital heart disease. The team of physicians looking after the neonate need to make a joint decision and cooperation amongst the specialities is mandatory. Cardiac status must be nearly optimal for a successful veno–venous bypass so that a veno–arterial bypass is preferred when cardiac function is compromised. Complex anatomical lesions may be repaired on ECMO, such as the repair of a laryngotracheal esophageal cleft, but where possible one wishes to defer repair until the child has been successfully weaned.

164 Ohm's law describes the relationship between current, resistance, and voltage. Each tissue type of the body has a characteristic resistance, which then dictates the amount of heat generated when a certain amount of current runs through that tissue. Therefore, the tissues that sustain the greatest amount of damage with electrical injury are conductive tissues of relatively high resistance. Most often (depending on the voltage, current, and other less tangible factors), the greatest damage occurs in muscles, especially where they narrow into tendons.

165–167: Questions

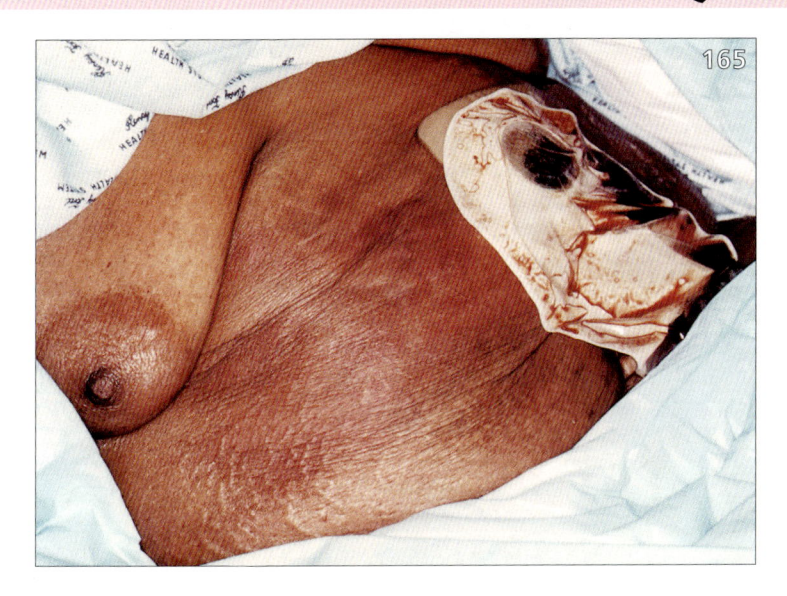

165 A 78-year-old female patient with diabetes mellitus, hypertension, and a previous stroke causing dysphagia, had a percutaneous gastrostomy placed. She presents 3 days later with abdominal pain, fever, and tachycardia. The skin examination is significant for crepitus on palpation and other signs (**165**).
i. What is the finding?
ii. What is the cause?
iii. What is the appropriate therapy?

166 A 69-year-old male with a past history of insulin-dependent diabetes mellitus and hypertension undergoes a right hemicolectomy for colon cancer. The parameters shown are obtained in the ICU. Calculate the systemic vascular resistance index.

HR 104/min
Systolic BP 140 mmHg (18.7 kPa)
Diastolic BP 90 mmHg (12.0 kPa)
CVP 16 mmHg (2.1 kPa)
Wedge pressure 11 mmHg (1.5 kPa)
Urine output 200 ml/hr
Cardiac index 2.5 l/min/m^2

167 A patient who is being treated with ampicillin for a cellulitis develops bloody diarrhea. The laboratory results reveal Gram-positive rods that grow anaerobically. The presence of a cytotoxin was demonstrated with the use of antibodies. What is the causative organism?

165–167: Answers

165 i. This patient presents with a necrotizing fasciitis, a deep seated infection of the subcutaneous tissue resulting in progressive destruction of fascia and fat. This is a very rare complication after percutaneous gastrostomy placement. The differentiation between cellulitis and fasciitis can be difficult in the early stages, but the presence of systemic symptoms and a rapid extension of the inflammatory process favors the necrotizing soft-tissue infection.

ii. The process is classically caused by group A streptococci or as in this case by a mixed bacterial flora consisting of anaerobes, Gram-negative aerobic bacilli, and enterococci. It has been associated with penetrating injuries, surgical procedures, diabetes mellitus, burns, and minor cuts.

iii. The administration of broad-spectrum antibiotics is not a sufficient therapy to cover this life-threatening complication. An emergency surgical consultation with prompt exploration and debridement is indicated.

166 In order to calculate the systemic vascular resistance, mean arterial blood pressure (MAP [mmHg]) must be calculated:

$$MAP = \frac{(SBP - DBP)}{3} + DBP$$

After calculation of the MAP the formula for systemic vascular resistance index can be used.

$$\frac{MAP - CVP \times 80}{CI}$$

The normal range for the systemic vascular resistance index is 1,600 to 2,400 dyne.sec cm^5/m^2. The systemic vascular resistance in this patient is 2,912 dyne.sec cm^5/m^2. Referring to the mathematic formula for the calculation of systemic vascular resistance an elevated resistance can be caused by a vasoconstriction, low preload or CVP and a low cardiac index. Depending upon the patient's condition one may choose to lower the systemic vascular resistance. Increasing the preload with fluid resuscitation, manipulating cardiac output with inotropic medications, or afterload reduction with vasodilators are all therapies which may provide benefit. One note of caution, vasodilation without adequate preload may cause hypotension.

167 *Clostridium difficile.*

168–170: Questions

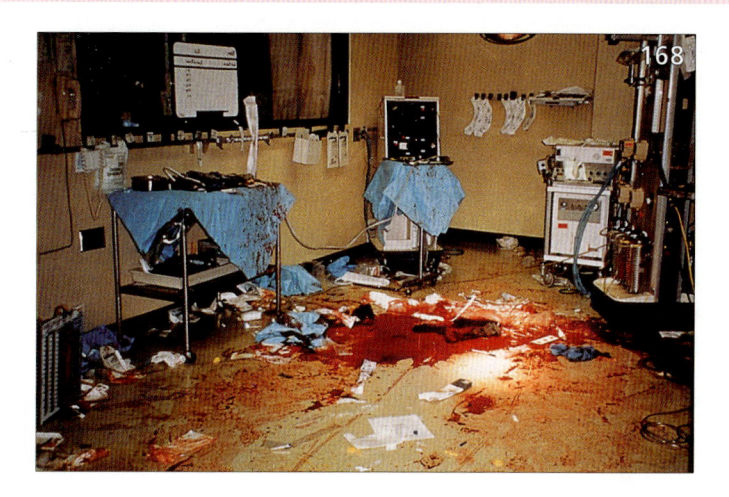

168 This is the scene following a resuscitative thoracotomy in an inner city trauma center (**168**).
i. What is the relative risk of contracting hepatitis or HIV from a blood transfusion?
ii. What is the relative risk of a health care professional getting hepatitis or HIV from a needle stick?
iii. What are the current recommendations should a health care worker receive an 'occupational exposure to the risk of HIV'?

169 A 32-year-old male pedestrian is struck by a motor vehicle, and suffers an open tibial fracture in the distal third of the lower leg. He is taken immediately to the operating room for debridement by the orthopedic surgeon. There is a heavily contaminated 5 × 5 cm (2 × 2 in) wound above the medial malleolus, and after pulse irrigation and debridement, a bone gap of 4 cm (1.6 in) is noted. Dorsalis pedis pulse is palpably normal. You are consulted for wound management. Which of the following steps are indicated?
A Placement of external fixator.
B Return to the operating room in 48 hours for redebridement.
C Immediate flap coverage.
D Plan for fasciocutaneous flap coverage.
E Plan for pedicled muscle flap coverage.
F Plan for free muscle flap coverage.

170 The best overall operative management of benign esophageal perforations is:
A Thoracotomy and drainage.
B Thoracotomy and resection.
C Exclusion and diversion.
D Thoracotomy and repair.
E Conservative management.

168–170: Answers

168 i. In the United States, the relative incidence of transfusion transmitted disease is as follows: hepatitis C 1:3,300; hepatitis B 1:200,000; HTLV 1:50,000; HIV 1:225,000. These refer to screened units of blood. In randomly tested members of the population, the incidence of HIV is 1:250. As many as 33% of inner city patients seen with penetrating trauma injuries are HIV positive.

ii. The risks of contracting hepatitis from an exposure are much greater than those of contracting HIV. One study suggested that the efficacy of HIV transmission is 0.3% (1:250), while that of hepatitis B virus from an hepatitis B antigen-positive patient ranges from 6–30%. The best preventive method includes use of universal precautions, using transfusions only for specific therapeutic endpoints, and avoiding needless blood exposure. Sharp instruments/needles should be handled in the following manner: do not recap needles; use disposable blades; cautery and scissors are better for dissection – do not pass sharp instruments directly, but rather use a 'neutral' zone; place needles and other 'sharps' in impervious containers.

iii. Should a health care worker be exposed to potentially infected HIV blood (e.g. needle stick, blood in the eye), current recommendations include serological testing of both the patient and the employee. If the patient is HIV positive, the health care worker should be tested for HIV and hepatitis B virus, the former at 0, 12 and 24 weeks. During the first 12 weeks the worker should avoid donating blood, sperm, and 'use safe sex practices'. Treatment has included prophylactic AZT, although this has not been definitely proven effective. It is more enthusiastically recommended if there has been a deep penetration or large volume of suspected contamination. Recommended regimes include that it be started within 72 hours, at 200 mg six times daily for 3 days, then 100–200 mg five times daily for the remainder of the month. Side effects include anemia, myalgia, and leukopenia. Because of teratogenic effects, effective birth control is required during treatment and for 4 weeks following completion; serological testing should be performed 1 year later because of the possibility of delayed conversion; women must not be pregnant or breast feeding.

169 A, B, and F. This patient has a severe contaminated combined bony and soft-tissue injury, and will benefit from a staged procedure. Placement of an external fixator for stabilization and subsequent serial debridement will verify which tissue will survive, and closure can be carried out when quantitative microbiology shows <100,000 organisms/g of tissue. Muscle provides the most well vascularized coverage, and in the distal third of the lower leg there are no good pedicled muscle flaps, therefore free tissue transfer is the best option.

170 D. The best overall approach for benign esophageal perforation without gross contamination or devitalization of tissue is to repair the esophagus. The treatment of esophageal perforation shows the mortality rate of 15% with primary repair, 34% with drainage alone, 29% with resection, 39% with exclusion and diversion, and 22% with nonoperative management. In the presence of an undilatable structure, however, the best treatment is resection with either immediate or interval reconstruction.

171–174: Questions

171 Discuss the diagnosis and management of a right ventricular infarct.

172 A 65-year-old male has undergone laparotomy for perforated diverticulitis with colon resection and end colostomy. One week later he still has spiking temperatures, persistent ileus, and elevated WBC count. Ongoing intra-abdominal sepsis is suspected. What would be the investigation of choice? What are the advantages and disadvantages of each radiologic modality?
A Ultrasound.
B CT scan.
C Plain films.
D Gastrointestinal contrast studies.

173 A 45-year-old male presents after a road traffic accident. He complains of mild abdominal pain, but is clinically stable. CT scans are obtained (**173a, b**). Discuss your management.

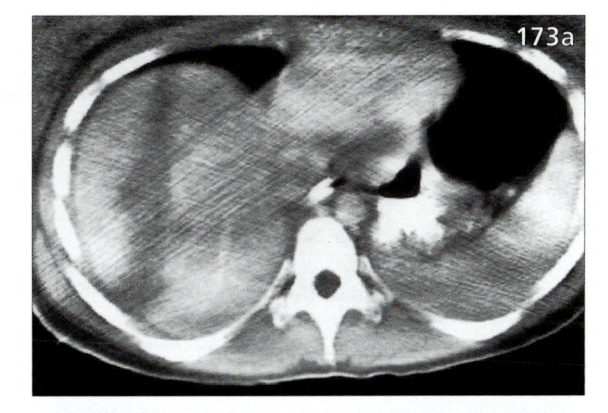

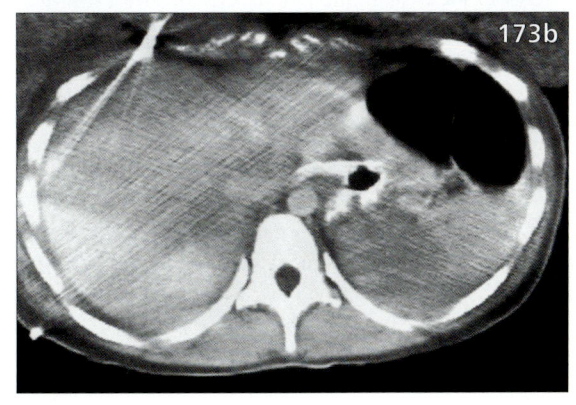

174 Anaphylaxis is:
A Mediated by IgM and IgE.
B A hypersensitivity type I reaction.
C Primarily involves T8 suppressor cells.
D Upregulation of T4 helper cells.
E Impossible in AIDS patients.

171–174: Answers

171 Isolated right ventricular myocardial infarction may be suggested by hypotension without pulmonary congestion. Evidence of inferior changes on ECG (II, III, VF) and jugular venous (JV) distension are confirmatory. Other important ECG changes are ST elevation in V4R (which should be done in all cases of cardiogenic shock) and Q waves and, or, ST elevation in V1–3 may also be suggestive. When right ventricular dysfunction is associated with shock, attempts should be made to maintain preload by volume resuscitation and avoiding vasodilators. If there is insufficient response (usually 1–2 l are required) dobutamine should be added. Pacemakers and early correction of atrial fibrillation may be required. Patients in shock should be considered for thrombolytic therapy or percutaneous transluminal coronary angioplasty.

172 A. Ultrasound is useful in assessing solid organs (liver, gall bladder, spleen, kidneys, uterus), subphrenic collections, subhepatic collections, and pelvic collections. Ultrasound cannot 'see through air' and thus loses utility in the setting of free air, persistent ileus, subcutaneous emphysema, or hyperinflated lungs. Advantages, however, include portability, noninvasiveness, and easy repeatability. B. A CT scan provides more information regarding the retroperitoneum. In the setting of ileus, intraperitoneal structures are better assessed. However, it necessitates both oral and IV contrast, which may be contraindicated in the septic ICU patient with deteriorating renal status. At times postoperative inflammatory findings, sterile collections, or nonopacified bowel are difficult to differentiate from postoperative abscesses. C. Plain films will demonstrate intestinal gas patterns, demonstrating ileus or obstruction. Generally an upright, supine, and lateral decubitus are obtained. Free air can be demonstrated on an upright or lateral decubitus film. Postoperatively free air may be visible up to 5 days, depending on the initial amount of free air and presence of adhesions. Clearly postoperative free air should rapidly decrease. Increasing amounts of free air give cause for alarm. In general, CT scans are more sensitive than plain films in detecting free air. D. Gastrointestinal contrast studies are of limited use in the postoperative setting. Ileus generally prevents forward propagation of upper gastrointestinal contrast. A perforated ulcer can be demonstrated. Lower gastrointestinal contrast studies are relatively contraindicated in the presence of recent lower bowel anastomoses. Although barium is contraindicated in the presence of perforation, it does provide better contrast, and is more sensitive in detecting perforations.

173 The CT scan demonstrates a transection of the liver and splenic hematoma with a small to moderate amount of fluid in the upper abdomen. The operative approach to the liver injury would be complicated and possibly could require right hepatectomy. With such a medial injury, there should be concern about possible inferior vena cava injury. If the patient is stable, without peritoneal changes, observation in a critical care unit, with serial hemoglobin determinations as well as bed rest, should be attempted. Early complications include bile leak, abscess, and continued bleeding.

174 B. Anaphylaxis is an immunological description of a type I hypersensitivity reaction mediated by IgE or IgG.

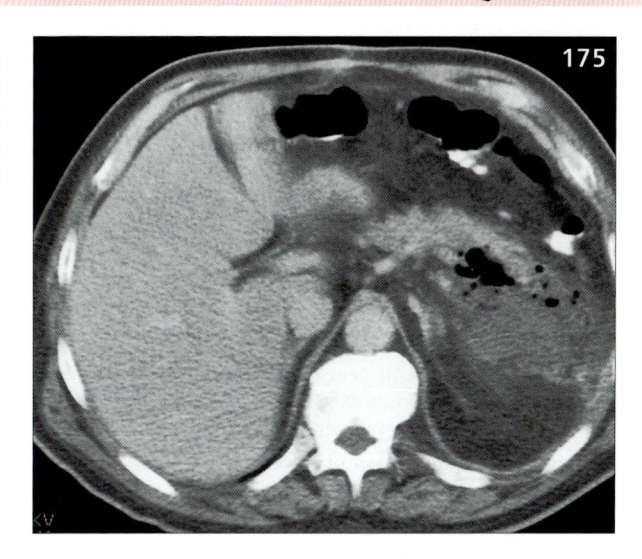

175–177: Questions

175 A patient with long history of ethanol abuse presents with fevers and abdominal pain. A CT is obtained (**175**). Discuss the management options.

176 A 30-year-old female is admitted to intensive care following a laparotomy for a massive postpartum hemorrhage. She has required 4 units of blood and 3,000 ml of crystalloid for volume resuscitation intraoperatively. However, she remains slightly hypotensive with a BP of 90/70 mmHg (12.0/9.3 kPa). Upon insertion of a pulmonary artery catheter introduced to aid in further fluid management, she desaturates to 80% suddenly becoming more tachycardic with bizarre ST and T wave changes on the ECG, tachypnea, and hypotension. What are the possible causes of this sudden event?

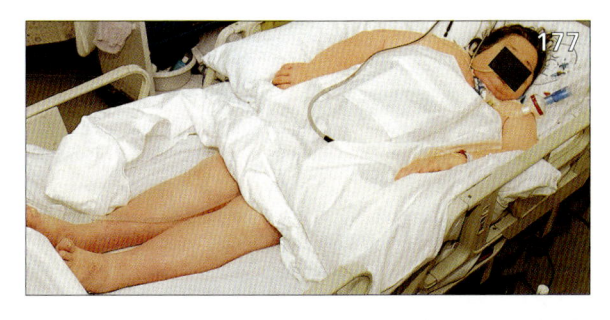

177 This 60-year-old female is a heavy smoker and 15 days ago had a laparotomy for a ruptured diverticulum with fecal soiling of her peritoneum (**177**). She became increasingly septic postoperatively and had a 'relook' laparotomy 3 days after her initial surgery at which her abdomen was irrigated and no septic focus was identified. She is now slowly recovering from her laparotomy and systemic inflammatory response syndrome. A percutaneous tracheostomy was inserted 5 days ago. She has minimal pulmonary secretions.
i. Is this patient ready to be weaned from the ventilator?
ii. List the reasons for your decision.

175–177: Answers

175 Infectious complications of pancreatitis may present with a range of CT findings from air bubbles to frank abscess. They require aggressive drainage and often operative debridement. This patient has a pancreatic abscess in the distal body/tail with fluid and air bubbles. This can be drained by percutaneous methods but may require operative drainage (which can be internal or external). Any evidence of infection on a CT scan in the setting of pancreatitis should be vigorously confirmed and treated.

176 Pulmonary embolism can be a devastating cause of profound sudden hypoxia. It is related to the most extreme of V/Q mismatches, namely a large section of ventilated lung without perfusion of blood, known as physiological respiratory dead space. Various substances can cause embolism and the profound cardiorespiratory effects are similar with venous thromboembolism, air embolism, and amniotic fluid embolism. Profound sudden hypoxia is the hallmark of pulmonary embolism which will be associated with tachypnea, a fall in end-tidal capnography trace, a raised CVP, and, if a pulmonary artery catheter is in place, high pulmonary artery pressures are often found. Auscultation of the chest is usually unremarkable in the acute setting. Cardiovascular changes can be equally dramatic with tachycardia and a dramatic fall in BP frequent. Much emphasis on ECG findings has been made in the past; however, the classical findings of right bundle branch block or S1, Q3, T3 are only found in <15% of cases, more often than not tachycardia with nonspecific ST segment and T wave changes are found. It is quite a difficult diagnosis to make in the acute setting but should be suspected by temporally related events, such as: recent diagnosis or treatment of deep vein thrombosis, proceeding central venous catheter placement (air embolism), recent delivery or cesarean section (amniotic fluid embolism), recent long bone fracture, or fixation of such a fracture with intramedullary reaming and nailing (fat embolism).

177 i. This lady is not ready to wean.
ii. There are a number of reasons for this. (1) She is very edematous. This has occurred as a result of the fluid therapy necessary to treat her sepsis. Her lungs are also highly likely to be edematous with ongoing protein leakage whilst she has an ongoing systemic inflammatory response syndrome. (2) She remains sedated. Sedation should be minimized to allow successful weaning. As the commonest cause of airway compromise is altered level of consciousness, then she needs to be awake enough to co-operate with the weaning process. (3) She is obese and lying supine. This combination is not ideal to minimize the work of her breathing. (4) She has a history of excess smoking, which may have progressed to chronic obstructive pulmonary disease further complicating her ability to come off a ventilator. A set of blood gases before her surgical admission would be invaluable to establish her normal levels of hypoxia or hypercarbia. Unfortunately, this is not commonly available. It could be difficult to wean her due to hitherto undetected long-standing respiratory insufficiency.

178–180: Questions

178 With regard to the patient in **177**, list the criteria that you would consider necessary before weaning from ventilation can be successful.

179 A 60-year-old male with known atrial fibrillation presents to the emergency room with a 7-hour history of right calf and foot pain which began suddenly. Physical examination reveals, a pulseless cool calf and foot with slow capillary refill and mild hypesthesia. Within the next hour the patient gets an arteriogram that shows an occlusion of his right common femoral artery bifurcation and otherwise normal vasculature. The patient undergoes an urgent right common femoral artery embolectomy and is transferred to the ICU with palpable distal pulses. Over the next 8 hours the right calf becomes progressively swollen and hard and the patient's urine is noted to become dark red in color. Now the pulses are barely audible with the continuous wave Doppler device. The most likely cause of these new findings is:
A Recurrent embolization to the right femoral artery.
B Compartment syndrome and myonecrosis.
C Acute thrombosis of the embolectomy site.
D Arterial spasm of the operated artery.

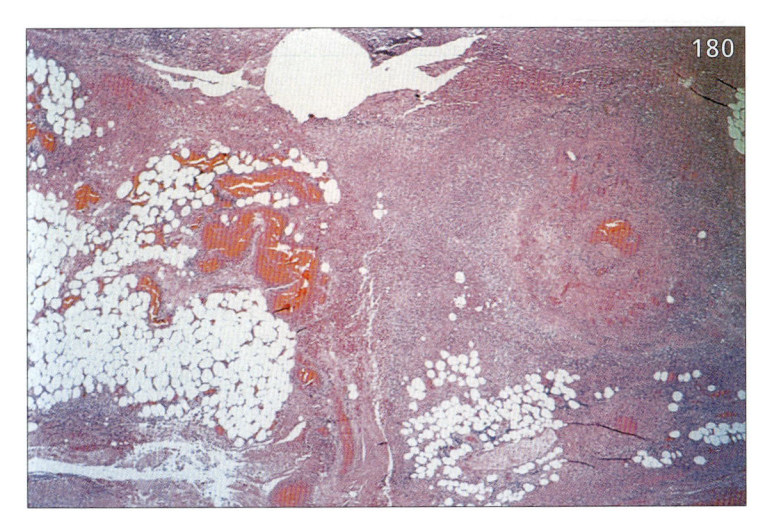

180 What are the histologic features of necrotizing soft-tissue infections (**180**)?

178–180: Answers

178 Criteria for successful weaning are: (1) Five minutes following cessation of positive pressure ventilation, the rapid shallow breathing index (respiratory rate (in breaths/min)/tidal volume (in litres)) should be checked and verified that it is <100. If >100 the patient is unlikely to cope with self-ventilation and therefore is not ready to be extubated/decannulated. (2) Evidence of increasing respiratory inco-ordination by observing the chest and abdomen is an indicator of possible failure to wean. (3) Evidence of increasing sympathetic drive (and potential hypercapnea or hypoxia) indicates failing ventilation. This can be suspected if the systolic blood pressure is rising (>20 mmHg (2.7 kPa) or 20%) or the pulse is rising to >100 beats/min (or by 20 beats/min or by 20%). (4) Arrhythmia development is further evidence of stress. (5) Oxygen saturation should not fall to <93%. (6) After 15 minutes and 30 minutes $PaCO_2$ should not rise by 20% (i.e. 7.5 mmHg (1 kPa)). (7) Conscious level should be maintained. Observe the patient continuously for signs of inco-ordination or tiredness, which almost invariably precedes blood gas evidence of fatigue. (8) Excessive amounts of pulmonary secretions make a successful wean unlikely. Sputum retention is not an indication of failure to wean, but suggests the need for physiotherapy. Inadequacy of coughing (power) suggests that weaning will fail. (9) Arterial blood gases should usually be measured (additionally) at 1, 2, 4 and 8 hours. This should be more frequent if observation suggests tiredness.

179 B. The patient has ischemia-reperfusion induced compartment syndrome and early myonecrosis. The patient should have emergent four compartment calf fasciotomies to relieve the increased intracompartmental pressure. Fasciotomies will improve the perfusion of the leg but will also produce additional reperfusion injury. The metabolic disorders associated with reperfusion are aggressively addressed. The most important of these derangements are: acidosis, hyperkalemia, myoglobinuria leading to acute renal failure, and pulmonary insufficiency secondary to washout of platelet aggregates and thrombotic debris from the revascularized leg.

180 The histologic features include intense leukocyte infiltration with microabscesses in the subcutaneous tissue, fascia, and potentially muscle layers. There is liquefaction and focal necrosis of these layers. Characteristically there is thrombosis of the microvasculature with nutrient vessel vasculitis and thrombosis. Gram stains of the tissue show the invading micro-organism.

181–183: Questions

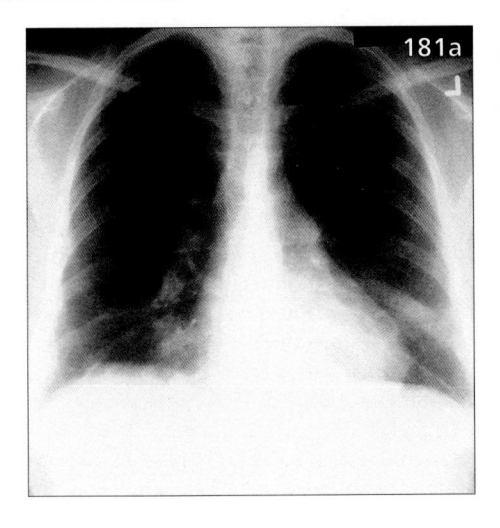

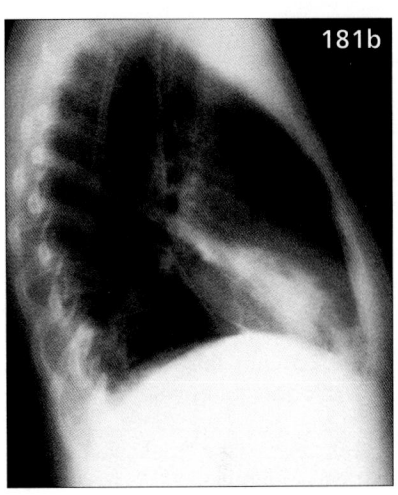

181 A 26-year-old prostitute, known to abuse intravenous drugs, presents with pneumonia caused by *Staphyloccocus aureus* infection. Chest X-rays (**181a, b**) show patchy bilateral pulmonary consolidation. She remains febrile despite 14 days of appropriate antibiotics. An echocardiogram is performed which shows large tricuspid vegetations. Discuss the further management of this patient.

182 Do these clinical conditions increase or decrease the SVO_2?
A Increasing FiO_2.
B Neuromuscular paralysis.
C Acute tension pneumothorax.
D Sepsis.
E Acute mesenteric ischemia.
F Ventilator disconnection.
G Arterial line disconnection.
H High dose vasopressors.
I Left ventricular failure.
J Shivering after blood transfusion.
K Ventricular septal defect after gunshot wound.
L Turning the patient.
M Presence of a fistula for a dialysis.

183 An intravenous drug abuser comes into the emergency room complaining of chest pain and shortness of breath. The patient states that a street doctor attempted a pocket shot and did not get a blood return for injection. His chest X-ray shows a small to moderate sized pneumothorax. What are your options for treatment in this patient?
A Do nothing.
B Catheter aspiration (CASP) tube.
C Chest tube.
D Thoracotomy.

181–183: Answers

181 Surgical intervention for tricuspid endocarditis is performed for severe embolic episodes, intractable CHF, persistent sepsis, or myocardial abscess. Many of these infections are caused by virulent organisms such as *S. aureus*, *Pseudomonas* species and fungi, all of which are difficult to eradicate with antibiotics alone. Because of this patient's failure to respond to a reasonable medical regimen, surgery would be indicated. A point of controversy exists when the patient is also HIV positive, where definitive benefit of surgery is lacking. Several surgical options exist, including simple valvectomy, valve debridement, and tricuspid valve replacement. Valvectomy is likely to be successful in the absence of pulmonary hypertension, although 20–30% will subsequently develop intractable right-sided failure. Debridement is not an alternative with annular or multileaflet involvement. Replacement risks prosthetic endocarditis, which is almost certainly fatal in these patients. The recurrence rate is high. This influences the dismal long-term results, with mortality rates of up to 90% at 5–10 years.

182 Because of the Fick equation relationships, an increase in SVO_2 implies an increase in cardiac output, a decrease in O_2 consumption, an increase in hemoglobin, or an increase in arterial oxygenation. Increasing the FiO_2, neuromuscular paralysis, sepsis, acute mesenteric ischemia, high dose vasopressors, a ventricular septal defect after a gunshot wound, and a fistula for a dialysis are all clinical conditions which serve to increase the SVO_2. A decreased SVO_2 is measured with acute tension pneumothorax, ventilator disconnection, hemorrhage from an arterial line disconnection, left ventricular failure, shivering after blood transfusion, and turning the patient. Conditions which decrease the cardiac output, increase the oxygen consumption, decrease hemoglobin or decrease arterial oxygenation are reflected in a decrease in SVO_2.

183 B and C. Pneumothorax size can be quantitated as small (<20% of total lung volume), moderate (20–40%) or large (>40%). Management of a small to moderate pneumothorax include both a CASP and chest tube (**183**). According to the Henry Ford Hospital's experience with 114 pneumothorax patients, the CASP tube is the less expensive and simpler alternative, especially for needle-induced or simple traumatic pneumothoraces (75% successful). The chest tube, however, remains the gold standard, especially for CASP failures and associated hemothorax or pleural effusion. In spontaneous pneumothoraces with large air leaks, tube drainage is required. Surgery is reserved for patients whose lungs do not expand using any of the other modalities

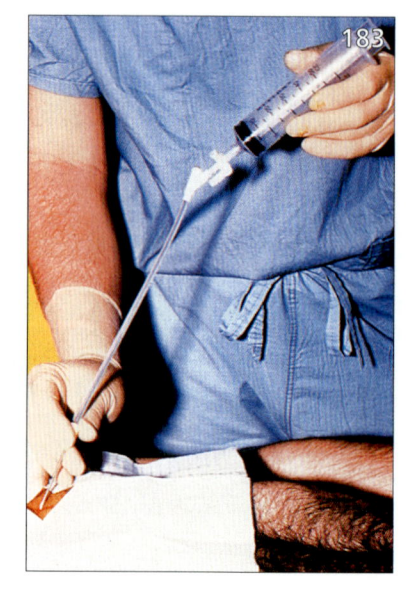

184–186: Questions

184 Discuss thrombolytic therapy in the management of acute myocardial ischemia.

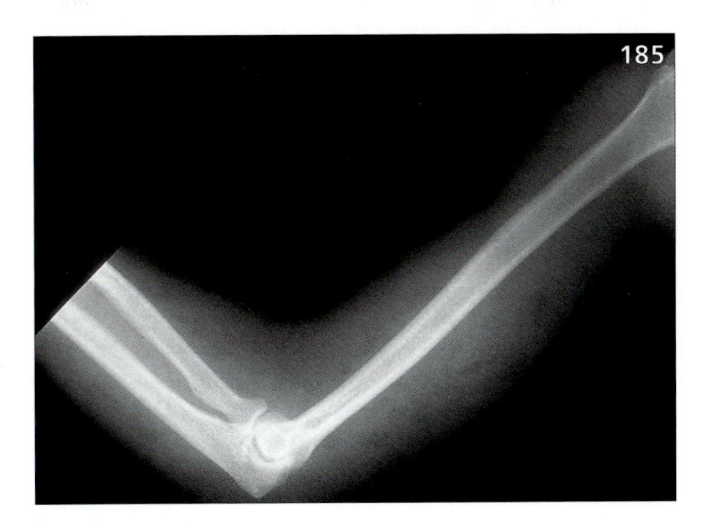

185 The radiograph (**185**) was obtained on a patient with a swollen forearm. Air is seen in the soft-tissue structures. What are the possible etiologies for this finding?

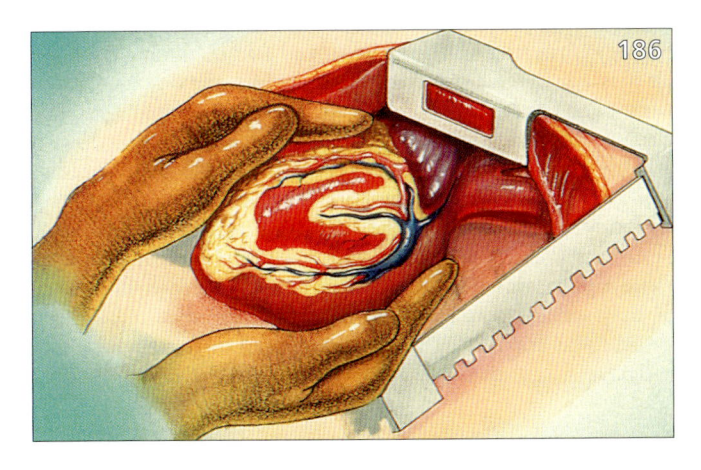

186 Discuss the indications for resuscitative thoracotomy in medical arrest (**186**).

184–186: Answers

184 When administered within 6 hours of signs and symptoms about 30 deaths/1,000 patients are prevented. When given between 7–12 hours, 20 deaths/1,000 patients are prevented. Streptokinase is administered as 1.5 million units in 100 ml dextrose and water or normal saline over 30–60 minutes. Anistreplase is given 30 units over 3–5 minutes. t-PA is given in 15 mg IV bolus, followed by 0.5 mg/kg over 60 minutes (maximum dose not >100 mg). Urokinase is given a 2 million units IV bolus or 1.5 million bolus and 1.5 million units over 1 hour. IV heparin for 48 hours appears to help improve coronary patency and survival with accelerated t-PA therapy (over 90 minutes rather than 3 hours) and urokinase. However, the activated partial thromboplastin time should be <90 seconds as greater values are associated with markedly increased risk of bleeding, including intracerebral. ASA (160–325 mg chewed) given acutely has an independent and additive benefit, and if maintained may result in reducing clinical events. Thrombolytic therapy results in about 3.9 strokes/1,000 patients treated (2/1,000 nonfatal). Risk factors include systolic hypertension and age over 75 years. Major noncerebral bleeds requiring transfusion or considered life threatening occur in 7/1,000 patients. Hypotension can occur following streptokinase and anistreplase, but major allergic reactions are rare. Routine corticosteroid use is not warranted as prophylaxis. Treatment usually involves temporary cessation of infusion, elevating the feet, and occasionally atropine or administering IV fluids.

185 Air in the soft-tissue plane of an extremity radiograph can be caused by a soft-tissue necrotizing infection, previous surgery with undermining of the skin and soft-tissue, peroxide irrigation, trauma, and extension of compressed gas with subcutaneous air from laparoscopic or thoracoscopic examinations or potentially in the upper extremities from extension of subcutaneous emphysema from the chest.

186 Indications for thoracotomy in medical arrests is controversial. Although the literature has demonstrated a greatly improved hemodynamic profile during open cardiac chest massage over closed chest compressions, the outcome has not improved in the human model. One reason is that open cardiac chest massage is not performed until closed chest compressions have failed which extends the downtime at least 20 minutes. One study found that the return of spontaneous circulation is time dependent and recommends that thoracotomy be done sooner (5 minutes after arrival to the emergency department) rather than later. The return of spontaneous circulation rate was highest in patients with early thoracotomy and declined as the timing of thoracotomy was delayed. Further study is needed to determine if open-chest cardiac massage, initiated concurrently with other advanced cardiac life support (ACLS) treatment, has any role in the management of medical cardiac arrests in select groups of patients.

187–189: Questions

187 A 20-year-old female arrives in the emergency department comatose with a Glasgow coma score of 8. No history is available. Vital signs are: BP 80/50 mmHg (10.7/6.7 kPa), HR 120/min, RR 30/min, temperature 38.5°C (101.3°F). Mucous membranes are dry. No neurologic localizing signs are present. The physical examination is otherwise noncontributory. Blood work is shown.

Hemoglobin 120 g/l (12.0 g/dl)	Creatine 150 µmol/l
WBC 18 × 10^9/l (18,000/mm^3)	(1.7 mg/dl)
Platelets 150 × 10^9/l (150,000/mm^3)	Plasma glucose 35 mmol/l
Na$^+$ 145 mmol/l (mEq/l)	(631 mg/dl)
K$^+$ 5.6 mmol/l (mEq/l)	pH 7.15 (H$^+$ 72)
Cl$^-$ 100 mmol/l (mEq/l)	PO_2 100 mmHg (13.3 kPa)
HCO$_3^-$ 10 mmol/l (mEq/l)	PCO_2 25 mmHg (3.3 kPa)
Urea 18 mmol/l (BUN 108 mg/dl)	

Her chest X-ray is normal. Preliminary urinalysis reveals 50 WBC/high power field with numerous Gram-negative organisms. How would you manage this patient?

188 A 44-year-old female presents to the emergency room with episodes of emesis. Initially these were bilious in nature but later turned bloody. The initial hemoglobin value is 115 g/l (11.5 g/dl). The patient is tachycardic on admission and gets admitted to the ICU. She admits to a history of intravenous heroin abuse and alcoholism. An esophagoduodenoscopy of the lower esophagus is shown (**188**).
i. Describe the finding?
ii. What is the etiology?
iii. What is the therapy and prognosis?

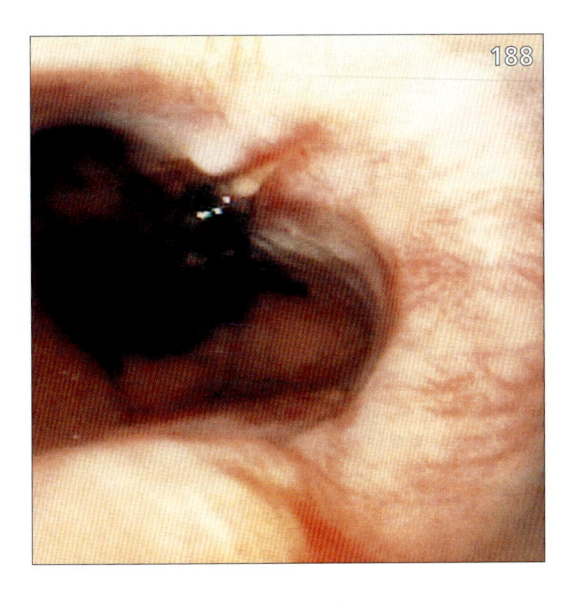

189 Discuss the management of microcirculatory thrombosis complicating a radial line.

187–189: Answers

187 Diabetic ketoacidosis often presents with severe dehydration, Kussmaul respirations, and depressed mentation. Plasma glucose is elevated as is anion gap. The anion gap is accounted for by elevated levels of ketone bodies. Total body potassium and phosphate levels are deplete, even though initial levels can be high. There is a small (<10%) mortality rate with diabetic ketoacidosis. Treatment involves aggressive volume replacement, electrolyte replacement (especially K^+ and P^{2+}), insulin administration (preferably by continuous drip, and not SQ/IM injections). Underlying medical precipitants need to be treated. For this patient, a urinary tract infection probably precipitated the diabetic ketoacidosis. Intubation is required for airway protection in cases of severe obtundation. Use of HCO_3^- is controversial. In general it is administered when severe acidosis is compromising cardiac status. Over aggressive fluid/electrolyte correction has been associated with cerebral edema. It is recommended that abnormalities be corrected over 24–48 hours, obviously more aggressively initially.

188 i. The patient has a mucosal tear (Mallory–Weiss lesion) in the lower esophagus with an adherent clot. These lacerations are common findings in patients undergoing endoscopy for upper gastrointestinal bleeding. They tend to occur more commonly in men than in women, usually in the third to fifth decade of life.
ii. Events that suddenly raise intra-abdominal pressure, such as emesis, seizures, hiccups or abdominal trauma can lead to Mallory–Weiss tears. Alcoholism has most frequently been associated with this entity. Hiatal hernias are frequently found and may constitute a risk factor. A rapid increase in intraluminal pressure during emesis that occurs in the intrathoracic location of the lower esophagus may induce the lesion.
iii. Most patients with Mallory–Weiss tears will stop bleeding spontaneously and do not need any further intervention. However, patients with evidence of ongoing bleeding will benefit from endoscopic intervention such as thermocoagulation, heater probe, or injection of epinephrine (adrenaline). Cases that fail this form of therapy need surgical intervention.

189 Microcirculatory thrombosis is treated by removing the line and treating the underlying problem. In the absence of low flow, the cause may be heparin induced thrombocytopenia. Thrombosis can result in ischemia and necrosis. Other successful therapies that have been tried include stellate ganglion blockade, surgical thrombectomy, and low dose thrombolytic agents. The risk of thrombosis can be lowered by insertion of the catheter in a vessel with abundant collaterals and flushing with heparin solution.

190–192: Questions

190 Describe how the steps indicated in the illustration (**190**) relate to the function of adrenergic and cholinergic receptors.

191 A 56-year-old male presents with a second episode this week of temporary weakness. He has had two previous myocardial infarctions and continues to have CCS class 3 angina. Carotid Doppler examination shows an occluded left internal carotid artery with a 90% stenosis of the right internal carotid. Discuss the further evaluation and management of this patient.

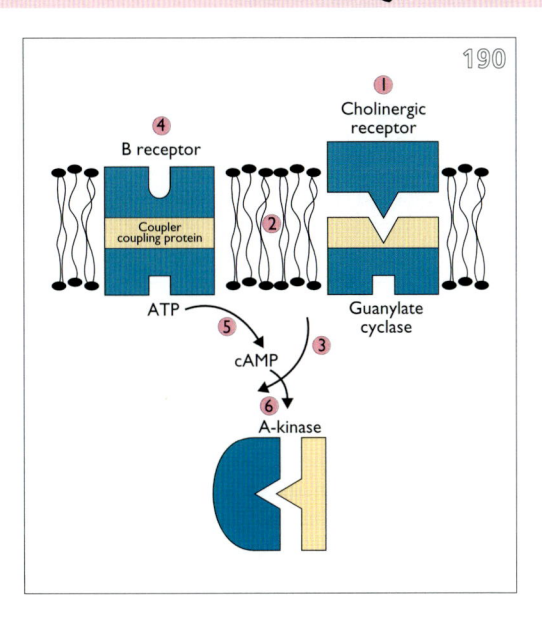

192 Are the following statements true or false?
A Acute lung injury is defined as $PaO_2/FiO_2 \leq 200$ mmHg (≤ 26.7 kPa), bilateral pulmonary infiltrates, PCOP ≤ 18 mmHg (≤ 2.4 kPa).
B ARDS is an acute lung injury with $PaO_2/FiO_2 \leq 300$ mmHg (≤ 40.0 kPa).
C Diffuse alveolar infiltrates are present immediately after the precipitating event in ARDS.
D The degree of lung involvement on chest CT correlates the gas exchange and compliance of the lung in ARDS.
E Initial ABGs show decrease PCO_2 and decrease PaO_2 in patients with ARDS.
F Increased protein content of the alveolar fluid indicates intact pulmonary alveolar capillary membranes.
G Measurement of extravascular lung water is a practical bedside test for ARDS.
H Large tidal volume ventilation is appropriate for patients with ARDS.
I PEEP is used to prevent ARDS.
J Permissive hypercapnia is used to decrease peak airway pressure in ARDS.
K Extracorporeal membrane oxygenation and extracorporeal CO_2 removal improve survival in ARDS.
L Nitric oxide produces decrease in pulmonary artery pressure and increases the PaO_2/FiO_2.
M Patients with ARDS do not benefit from high dose corticosteroids.
N Ibuprofen, indomethacin, acetylcysteine and ketoconazole are effective agents for treatment of ARDS.

190–192: Answers

190 (1) Acetylcholine binds to the outer protein of the cholinergic receptor. This activates the inner protein, guanylate cyclase, stimulating the conversion of GTP to cGMP, which in turn: (2) blocks the coupler protein in the adrenergic receptor and (3) blocks the interaction of cAMP with A-kinase. (4) The beta-adrenergic receptor consists of three proteins: an outer receptor; a middle coupler protein which stimulates the conversion of GTP to GMP and also stimulates the inner protein, adenylate cyclase. This protein in turn acts to: (5) convert ATP to cAMP which then: (6) activates A-kinase. A-kinase phosphorylate regulatory proteins of the actin-myosin complex, Ca^{2+} channels and Ca^{2+} pumps on the sarcoplasmic reticulum as well as on the membrane. The net result is an increase in intracellular Ca^{2+} concentration, an increased clearance of calcium, and increased sensitivity to calcium by the contractile proteins. This is the basis of the inotropic and chronotropic effects of adrenergic stimulating agents.

191 The simultaneous presence of symptomatic cerebrovascular disease and coronary artery disease presents a therapeutic dilemma: should one lesion be addressed before the other or both together? If the carotid disease is tackled first, the patient may suffer a myocardial infarction and if the coronaries are addressed first, a stroke might occur. If addressed simultaneously, the morbidity of each procedure is combined. A reasonable approach is to address the most symptomatic lesion first. If both are very symptomatic, then a combined procedure should be planned.

This patient requires angiography of his cerebral and coronary circulations, as well as an assessment of ventricular function and general medical status. As both lesions are very symptomatic, a simultaneous operation should be planned. A sensible operative approach is to first open the chest and make all the precardiopulmonary bypass preparations including harvesting of conduit, opening the pericardium, and placement of aortic and atrial pursestring sutures. After this the carotid endarterectomy may be undertaken (probably using a shunt in this instance), instituting cardiopulmonary bypass only in the event of hemodynamic instability. Another approach would be to institute cardiopulmonary bypass with hypothermia before performing the endarterectomy followed by coronary artery bypass during the rewarming period. No randomized data exist to further clarify this controversial area.

192
A False.
B False.
C False.
D True.
E True.
F False.
G False.
H False.
I False.
J True.
K False.
L True.
M True.
N False.

193–196: Questions

193 A 69-year-old male with symptomatic 80% stenosis of his left internal carotid artery undergoes an uneventful carotid endarterectomy under general anesthesia. Two hours following the conclusion of the operation the patient arrives in the ICU awake and talking. When examined 30 minutes later he is found to be aphasic with a right hemiparesis. How would you manage this problem?
A Obtain an urgent arteriogram.
B Obtain a CT scan of the head.
C Return the patient to the operating room for immediate re-exploration.
D Start IV heparin and request an urgent neurological consultation.

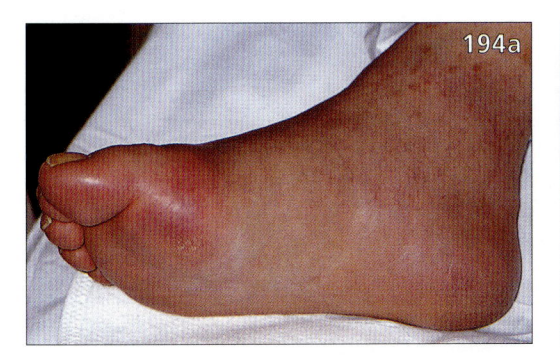

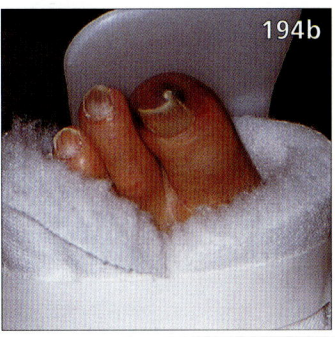

194 Match the photograph of the foot to the clinical condition (**194a, b**).
A Trash foot or blue toe syndrome.   B Continued hypotension from sepsis.

195 Match the drug (A–D) to the effect (1–8).
A Aspirin.
B Warfarin.
C Heparin.
D t-PA.

1 Dermal necrosis.
2 Inhibits cyclo-oxygenase.
3 Lysis clot.
4 Thrombocytopenia.
5 Bound to albumin.
6 Increases fibrin degradation products.
7 Inhibits thromboxin A_2 synthesis.
8 Vitamin K antagonist.

196 Microscopic examination of a tissue sample sent for analysis reveals yeasts and pseudohyphae. The organism produces Gram-positive colonies on Sabouraud's agar. It forms chlamydospores. What is the organism?

193–196: Answers

193 C. The patient developed an acute ischemic episode in the immediate postoperative period which is most likely secondary to thrombosis of the operated internal cartoid artery. In this case, the diagnosis of the stroke is made by physical examination and the patient should return to the operating room for re-exploration in an effort to re-establish circulation to the ischemic part of the brain. The best results from reoperation are usually reported when blood flow is restored within 1–2 hours from the onset of symptoms. The team caring for the patient should not, therefore, delay his return to the operating room to obtain any further diagnostic tests.

194 Photograph **194b** demonstrates the trash foot or blue toe syndrome. The lesions are demarcated and usually involve individual toes. Most commonly this is associated with distal embolization from central atherosclerotic plaques on the aorta. Any emboli originating centrally (including the heart) can produce this syndrome. This can occur following aortic surgery, aortic angiography, or intra-arterial injection related to intravenous drug abuse. Treatment is generally supportive, although various peripheral vasodilators have been tried. Photograph **194a** is of a patient who is hypotensive. This foot is generally cold and clammy. It has delayed capillary refill and a pale appearance. This reflects an under-resuscitated septic patient who has clamped down peripherally and to the soft tissue in order to conserve volume centrally.

195 A. The chief effect of aspirin is its effect on cyclo-oxygenase and subsequent inhibition of thromboxin A_2 synthesis. This effects takes place directly in the platelet throughout its life span. This alters platelet adhesion, but does not cause thrombocytopenia. B. The chief action of warfarin is the inhibition of factors VII, II, IX, and X, and protein. The above mentioned factors are the vitamin K dependent factors, so that warfarin is a vitamin K antagonist. Warfarin is bound to plasma albumin and only the free warfarin is biologically active. Decreased albumin levels, and drugs that compete with the warfarin binding on albumin, alter the amount of free drug available to act as an anticoagulant. Multiple skin reactions are seen with warfarin. These include bleeding into the skin with ecchymoses and purpura. Dermal necrosis is a very rare complication of warfarin therapy which begins as the formation of a rash, progressing to hemorrhagic bullae and skin sloughing. C. Heparin interferes with blood coagulation through actions in conjunction with antithrombin III. Approximately 6% of patients develop thrombocytopenia during their second week of heparin therapy. D. t-PA has fibrinolytic activity and causes clot lysis. It works through the enhanced activation of plasminogen. As the clot breaks down, fibrin degradation products are formed.

196 *Candida albicans.*

197–200: Questions

197 A hypothetical burn (**197a**) on a 70 kg (155 lb) patient. Using the Lund–Browder chart (**197b**), determine the percentage of second and third degree burns on the patient, and write fluid orders for the first 24 hours based on your calculation.

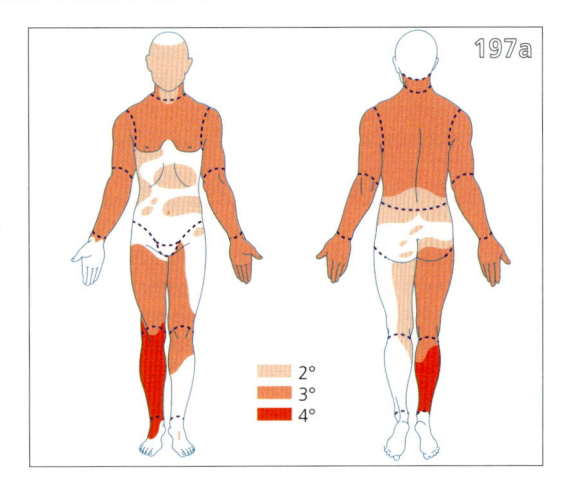

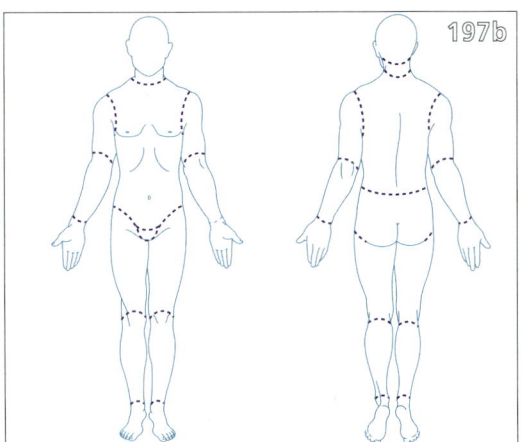

198 A pulmonary artery catheter is placed in a patient in the ICU and no wave form is displayed on the scope. What is the cause of this problem?

199 A vehicle carrying several containers of propane rolls over several times on a still, cold fall morning. The driver was trapped inside. Discuss the initial approach that emergency services personnel should take.

200 i. Is sepsis or inhalation injury the most important cause of fire-related deaths?
ii. What is the gold-standard method to make the diagnosis of inhalation injury?
iii. What are corollary indications of inhalation injury?

141

197–200: Answers

197 Use the Lund–Browder chart (all areas are multiples of 9, except groin – 1%). This severe burn represents 16% of the total body surface area for second degree and 68% the total body surface area for third degree. A total of 84% of the total body surface area involvement (TBSA) is used for the calculation by Parkland formula:

(% body surface area burn)(4)(body weight (kg)) = ml in 24 hours.

In this case, 23,520 ml of crystalloid is required in 24 hours. Half of the volume (11,760 ml) is given in the first 8 hours. NB: This amount needs to be before 8 hours have passed after the injury, and if it took the patient 7 hours to get to you, all of it is supposed to be delivered in the remaining hour. The balance of 11,760 ml is then given in the remaining 16 hours. It is important to remember that this calculation is a first approximation, and mid-course corrections need to be made depending on the patient's physiologic response.

198 Possible causes are incorrect stop-cock position, clots in the catheter, problems with the transducer dome including entrapped air, incorrect connection of the transducer, or a defective transducer. The final problem may include improper calibration.

199 The first task of all rescue personnel is to assess and control the scene. In this case the propane, cooled by the ambient temperature, had formed a clear cloud around the vehicle. In this setting, a spark or flame could cause a fire or explosion. The first task is, therefore, to control the site. The driver was removed by rapid extraction techniques after the fire department crew dissipated the cloud using 'attack and support' lines.

200 i. Inhalation injury remains the leading cause of death after fire. Sepsis is the second most common cause of mortality.
ii. The basis of a firm diagnosis of inhalation injury remains bronchoscopy, with evidence of bronchial soot and erythema.
iii. Corollary indications of inhalation injury include a history of fire in a closed space, singeing of facial hairs, hoarseness, cough, stridor, and erythema and edema of the upper aerodigestive tract.

201–203: Questions

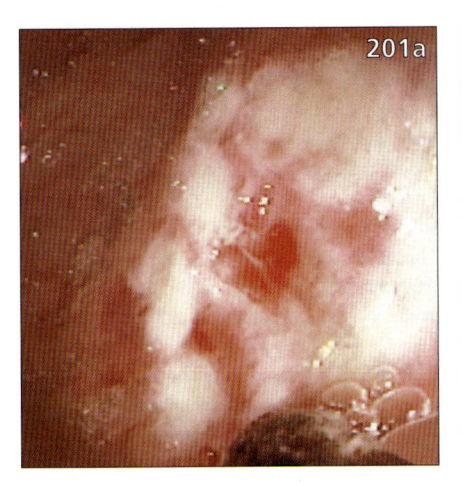

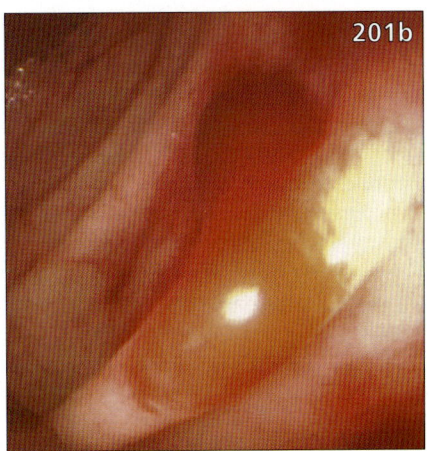

201 A 59-year-old male is admitted to the hospital with hematochezia. He denies abdominal pain, nausea, emesis, or hematemesis. At first, he had noticed blood mixed in with some stool, later he saw frank blood. He does not take any NSAIDs or ASA. There is no other significant medical or surgical history. His hemoglobin on admission was found to be 98 g/l (9.8 g/dl).
i. What is your initial diagnosis?
ii. How would you proceed with a diagnosis?
iii. Endoscopy of the cecum reveals these pictures (**201a, b**). What is your diagnosis?

202 Discuss the role of sodium bicarbonate administration in cardiac arrest or shock.

203 Which statement regarding mechanical ventilation in status asthmaticus is true?
A Muscle paralysis with a nondepolarizing neuromuscular agent decreases chest wall compliance.
B High minute ventilation generates low peak airway pressures.
C PEEP increases cardiac output in patients with status because of high airway resistance.
D Mucus plugging can be avoided with a high dose of corticosteriods.
E End-inspiratory lung volumes increase with a decrease in expiratory times.

201–203: Answers

201 i. The patient presents with hematochezia, suggestive of a lower gastrointestinal bleeding. In a substantial number of cases, however, an upper gastrointestinal bleeding can present in this manner. The first goal in any patient presenting with an acute bleeding should be evaluation of the hemodynamic parameters and subsequent stabilization. A nasogastric tube with lavage should be placed. A negative lavage does not rule out the possibility of a postbulbar ulcer with bleeding. In the absence of postural hypotension, negative nasogastric aspirate, and no prior ulcer or medication associated with ulcers, an upper gastrointestinal tract source becomes less likely. A source in the colon or small bowel is likely. The major differential diagnosis includes diverticular bleeding, angiodysplasia of the colon, ischemic colitis, and neoplastic lesions in the colon.
ii. The only way to rule out an upper gastrointestinal tract source for a patient with hematochezia is to proceed with a esophagogastroduodenoscopy. Patients with a significant blood loss may not be safely studied by endoscopy and should proceed with an angiography to localize the source of bleeding. Otherwise, the patient needs a colonoscopic evaluation after preparation. Barium studies are not optimal to define mucosal lesions and also do not offer any therapeutic advantage.
iii. The lesion here is a vascular ectasis (angiodysplasia). This lesion most commonly presents with a low grade bleeding or iron deficiency anemia. In approximately 15% it shows a significant hemorrhage. The initial step is always a careful examination of the mucosa during a colonoscopy. Lesions that are found incidentally are best left alone, since the natural history of vascular ectasias supports that. Lesions that are actively bleeding or that have bled need intervention. Among endoscopic procedures currently used are laser ablation, bipolar thermocoagulation, and heater probe. If this therapy is not successful angiography with embolization can be used but preferably a right hemicolectomy is indicated. In 10–20% rebleeding can be encountered.

202 The treatment of acidosis with sodium bicarbonate is somewhat controversial. In patients with cardiac arrest with no real effective cardiac output, it is thought that sodium bicarbonate may actually be harmful. This is because the pH from ABGs is not reflective of venous and thus intracellular acidosis. Administration of bicarbonate may result in increased cellular acidosis and a worsening of cellular dysfunction. The acidosis should be treated by improving perfusion and ventilation. Following the restoration of spontaneous circulation, careful use of bicarbonate may be appropriate and when tissue perfusion, ventilation, and, or, oxygenation are inadequate, it appears that the routine use of bicarbonate may have negative effects on cellular and organ system function.

203 E. Muscle paralysis increases chest wall compliance. High minute ventilation generates high peak airway pressures because airway resistance is already high in these patients while PEEP decreases cardiac output. Mucus plugging is treated with vigorous pulmonary toilet. End-inspiratory lung volumes increase with a decrease in expiratory times causing pulmonary hyperinflation. Pulmonary hyperinflation can be avoided by allowing adequate time for exhalation.

204, 205: Questions

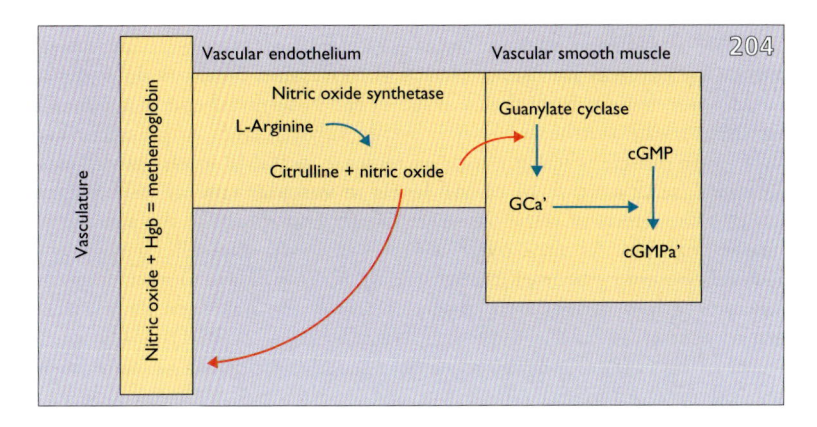

204 The diagram (**204**) depicts the pharmacologic pathway of nitric oxide in the pulmonary vasculature.
i. Describe the anticipated pulmonary effects of inhalational nitric oxide.
ii. What concentrations are thought to be effective in the treatment of ARDS?
iii. What are the primary toxicity concerns with the administration of nitric oxide?

205 Match the signs (A–I) with the descriptions (1–9):
A Homan's sign.
B Abraham's sign.
C Claybrook's sign.
D Grey–Turner's sign.
E Ewart's sign.
F Kussmaul's sign.
G Musset's sign.
H Drummond's sign.
I Trousseau's sign.

1 Pain in the back of the knee or calf when the ankle is dorsiflexed (with the knee bent), seen with deep venous thrombosis.
2 Rales, adventitious sounds, or dullness over the acromial end of the clavicle, seen with upper lobe tuberculosis.
3 Transmission of breath and heart sounds through the abdominal wall associated with a ruptured viscous.
4 Discoloration around the umbilicus, seen in retroperitoneal hemorrhage, especially hemorrhage pancreatitis.
5 An area of dullness with bronchial breath sounds appreciated below the left scapula, seen in large pericardial effusions with consequent lung compression.
6 Paradoxic increase in venous distension during inspiration, seen in cardiac tamponade.
7 Rhythmic head bobbing synchronous with the heart beat, seen in severe aortic insufficiency.
8 A puffing sound, synchronous with cardiac systole, heard from the nostrils when the mouth is closed, seen with aortic aneurysm.
9 Carpopedal spasm when the upper arm is compressed by a tourniquet or blood pressure cuff, seen in tetany.

204, 205: Answers

204 i. In 1987 endothelial relaxing factor was identified as nitric oxide and demonstrated to be the pathway for agents such as nitroprusside. Nitric oxide is produced in the vascular endothelium from the cleavage of the N-terminal end of arginine by the enzyme nitric oxide synthetase. Nitric oxide subsequently migrates to adjacent vascular smooth muscle where it effects an increase in cGMP levels via stimulation of guanylate cyclase. Elevation of cGMP levels in vascular smooth muscle produces vasodilation. The effects of nitric oxide are locally limited due to the affinity of nitric oxide for hemoglobin. As nitric oxide migrates from the intracellular environment it is immediately bound by hemoglobin with resultant conversion to methemoglobin.

ii. At extremely low doses (5–50 p.p.b.) nitric oxide has been demonstrated to improve oxygenation and reduce venous admixture (Qva/Qt). The presumed mechanism of this effect is by direct, local vasodilation of the vasculature serving ventilated alveoli. At higher concentrations (1–30 p.p.m.) nitric oxide has been demonstrated to reduce pulmonary artery hypertension. This effect is particularly important in advanced ARDS where significant pulmonary artery hypertension often produces right ventricular dysfunction.

iii. The potential toxicity of nitric oxide remains to be demonstrated. The North American Nitric Oxide Study Group (NIOSH) permits exposure to nitric oxide at 25 p.p.m. for up to 8 hr/day. Therapeutic levels of inhalational nitric oxide are in the range of 1–40 p.p.m. High levels of nitric oxide (5,000–20,000 p.p.m.) are associated with hypoxemia and death. The primary toxicity concern with nitric oxide relates to the generation of methemoglobin and nitric dioxide. Most clinical investigations have documented methemoglobin levels of <5 p.p.m. when nitric oxide concentrations are below 40 p.p.m. Nitric dioxide is produced when nitric oxide is exposed to oxygen. Nitric dioxide is relatively toxic and exposure is limited to <5 p.p.m. by NIOSH. The generation of nitric dioxide may be controlled by limiting circuit time and through the use of lime soda scrubbers. The use of these precautions has limited the measurable nitric dioxide levels to <1 p.p.m.

205 A and 5.
B and 3.
C and 2.
D and 6.
E and 9.
F and 7.
G and 4.
H and 1.
I and 8.

206–208: Questions

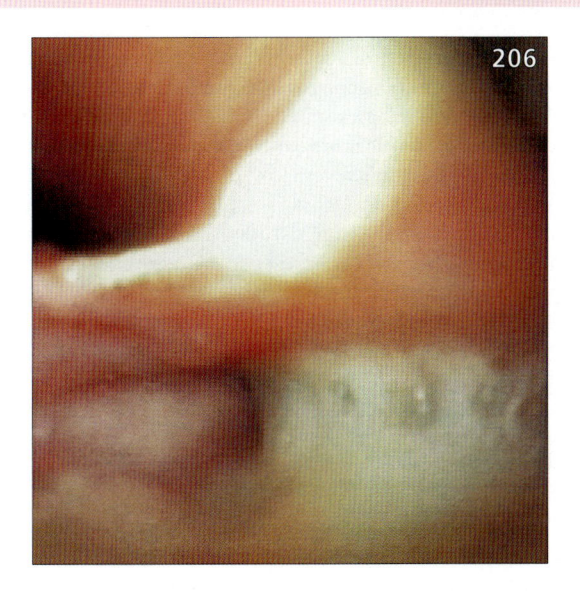

206 A 64-year-old male with a history of squamous cell carcinoma of his thoracic esophagus presents 6 months after completion of chemo- and radiation therapy with dysphagia and two episodes of left lower lobe pneumonia. An esophagoscopy reveals the finding shown (**206**).
i. What is the abnormality seen?
ii. What other modalities can be used to diagnose this condition?
iii. How would you treat this patient?

207 A 45-year-old male is brought to the emergency department in cardiac arrest. CPR is begun and the patient is intubated. An end-tidal CO_2 monitor is attached to the end of the ET tube. Chest compressions are constant a a rate of 72/min and a depth of 5 cm (2 in). Ventilation is delivered at a rate of 12/min in a six-compression-to-one-ventilation duty cycle. The end-tidal CO_2 ($PetCO_2$) is 15 mmHg (2.0 kPa). Discuss the end-tidal CO_2 monitoring during cardiac arrest and its predictive value of return of spontaneous circulation.

208 Match the drug (A–D) with its side effect (1–4):
A Hydralazine.
B Esmolol.
C Enalapril.
D Nitroprusside.

1 Angioedema.
2 Bronchospasm.
3 Tachycardia.
4 Metabolic acidosis.

206–208: Answers

206 i. The picture shows a large tracheoesophageal fistula (approximately 2 cm [1 in] in size), extending from the mid-esophagus into the bifurcation of the trachea.
ii. In cases of a suspected tracheoesophageal fistula, the procedure of choice is a barium swallow study. Water-soluble contrast material could cause pulmonary edema and respiratory distress, however, low osmolality water-soluble material can be used safely. Another imaging modality is a CT scan of the chest, which may not demonstrate small tracheoesophageal fistulas, but has the additional benefit of demonstrating mediastinal structures, presence of lymphadenopathy, and possible hepatic involvement of the primary tumor.
iii. A prosthesis is the therapy of choice to palliate a tracheoesophageal fistula. Newer types of stents which are self-expandable metal devices with coating can avoid some of the disadvantages of plastic prosthesis, such as perforation and migration. Before the deployment, the esophagus needs to be dilated sufficiently and there should be at least 2 cm (0.8 in) distance between the stent and the upper esophageal sphincter to avoid cervical dysphagia.

207 The concentration of expired CO_2 is a result of alveolar ventilation, pulmonary blood flow, and production of CO_2. Measurement of end-tidal CO_2 by either infrared absorption or mass-spectrophotometric techniques reflects pulmonary blood flow and cardiac output. After cardiac arrest, a marked decrease of cardiac output and thus pulmonary blood flow occurs. Correspondingly, a decrease in end-tidal CO_2 follows. One clinical study found that end-tidal CO_2 monitoring during CPR could be used as a prognostic indicator of resuscitation and survival. Thirty-five cardiac arrests were studied. Nine patients who were successfully resuscitated had higher average end-tidal CO_2 than those who were not resuscitated (15 mmHg versus 7 mmHg (2.0 kPa vs 0.9 kPa)). No patient with an average end-tidal CO_2 of <10 mmHg (1.3 kPa) was resuscitated.

208 A and 3; B and 2; C and 1; D and 4. Hydralazine is a potent arterial vasodilator. Hydralazine increases cardiac output and HR with the major side effects of tachycardia and headaches. This drug must be used with caution in patients with angina, myocardial infarction, and aortic dissection. Esmolol is a beta$_1$ selective beta blocker which has a very short duration of action. Severe hypotension is the most common adverse side effect seen; however, in patients with bronchospastic disease because this is a beta$_1$ selective blocker, it can increase bronchospasm. Enalapril is a potent ACE inhibitor. Severe hypotension is the most common adverse side effect seen. Patients receiving this medication can develop angioedema. Nitroprusside is a vasodilator. Nitroprusside is metabolized to thiocyanate. Toxicity symptoms are mental status changes, nausea, abdominal pain, tinnitus, hyperreflexia, and seizures. Cyanide toxicity can also occur and is manifested by metabolic acidosis, shortness of breath, headache, vomiting, dizziness, and loss of consciousness. Cyanide toxicity may also be associated with absent reflexes, dilated pupils, and a pink color.

209, 210: Questions

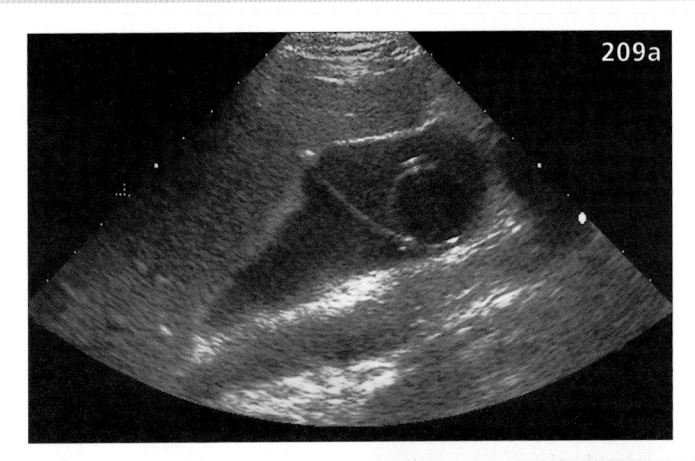

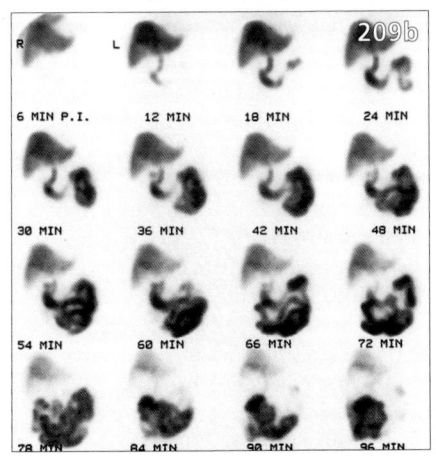

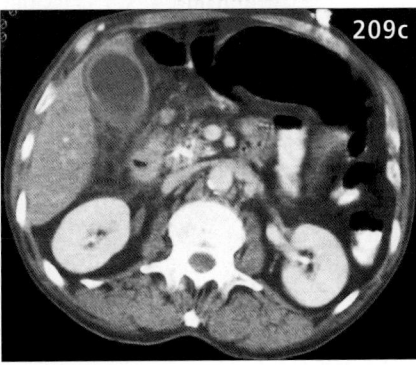

209 A 72-year-old male in the ICU following subarachnoid hemorrhage develops mild fever, elevated WBC count, high gastric residuals, and jaundice. Radiographs are shown (**209a–c**). Discuss the management options under the following circumstances:
A He is alert, extubated, and is stable.
B He is obtunded, ventilator dependent, and neurologic outcome is grim.
C He is febrile, had evidence of disseminated intravascular coagulation and sepsis.
D He has low grade fevers, but also evidence of vasospasm requiring aggressive treatment. There are no coagulation abnormalities.

210 i. Which patients benefit from continuous modes of dialysis?
ii. What are CAVH, CAVHD, SCUF, CVVH, CVVHD, and CVVHDF?
iii. What advantage does each modality have?

209, 210: Answers

209 Acalculous cholecystitis is difficult to diagnose. It may present with vague signs and symptoms including positive blood cultures demonstrating enteric bacteria, decreased intestinal and gastric motility, and frank cholangitis. Ultrasound, nuclear studies, and CT scans are all helpful but may not be conclusive. In high risk patients with some clinical evidence to suggest the diagnosis, percutanous drainage can be diagnostic and therapeutic. Because the technique involves going through the liver parenchyma to secure the tube, coagulation parameters must be normal. The management under the circumstances given should be: A. Cholecystectomy, can be done relatively electively. B. Percutaneous drainage. C. Open drainage or cholecystectomy depending on overall condition. D. Percutaneous drainage.

210 i. Intermittent modes of dialysis include hemodialysis and peritoneal dialysis.
ii. Continuous renal replacement options are: CAVH Continuous arteriovenous hemofiltration. CAVHD Continuous arteriovenous hemodiafiltration. SCUF Slow continuous ultrafiltration. CVVH Continuous venovenous hemodialysis. CVVHD Continuous venovenous hemodiafiltration. CVVHDF Continuous venovenous hemodialysis with filtration.
iii. Hemodialysis is indicated for patients with renal failure, fluid balance concerns, or metabolic concerns. In the presence of cardiovascular instability, continuous modes of dialysis are preferred. CAVH is driven by the patient's own BP. Blood is ultrafiltrated with convection transfer of molecules. Arterial and venous cannulation are required. As solutes are only removed by convection, adequate clearance may not be achieved. Fluid removal is variable. CAVHD is similar to CAVH but involves countercurrent dialysis as well. Clearance is increased by diffusion. Blood flow through the filter is controlled by the patient's BP. Fluid removal rates may vary. SCUF removes fluid by ultrafiltration only. Solutes are removed by convection. Fluid removal can be controlled. CVVH is slow continuous ultrafiltration with convection transfer of molecules. Blood flow and fluid removal are controlled by a pump. A dual lumen venous catheter is required. Improved clearance of middle molecules is obtained. CVVHD allows both ultrafiltration and diffusion solute clearance. Counter current dialysis is added to CVVH. Fluid removal is controlled. Electrolyte abnormalities can be corrected. Waste products (small molecules) are removed. CVVHDF involves use of a prefilter replacement solution, which enhances clearance. CVVHD and CVVHDF have become the continuous dialysis therapies of choice.

The disadvantages of CVVHD in comparison to intermittent hemodialysis include the need for anticoagulation and increased cost. Data regarding drug clearance in continuous modes of dialysis is slowly accumulating. Advantages of continuous dialysis modes over intermittent hemodialysis include improved patient tolerance, slow fluid removal, avoidance of rapid electrolyte shifts, and minimal need for volume restriction.

211–214: Questions

211 A chest CT of a patient who required ventilation because of progressive respiratory failure is shown (**211a**). After intubation it was noted that there was progressively increasing airway pressures with continued hypercapnia. What maneuvers could be tried?

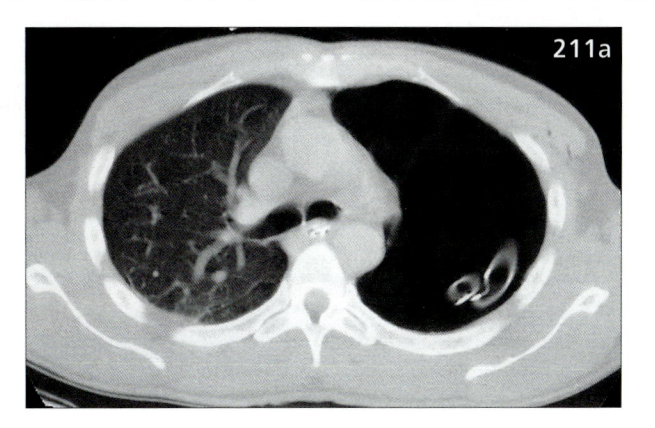

212 A 37-year-old male with chronic renal failure is admitted for gastrointestinal bleeding. He is diagnosed to have colonic angiodysplasia; surgical resection is planned. Preoperative bowel preparation includes soap suds enemas and oral magnesium nitrate. On the day of surgery, the patient is hyporeflexic, weak, sedated, with a blood pressure of 110/70 mmHg (14.7/9.3 kPa). Laboratory analysis is shown. What is the most likely cause?

Na^+	137 mmol/l (mEq/l)
K^+	4.1 mmol/l (mEq/l)
Cl^-	105 mmol/l (mEq/l)
CO_2	18 mmol/l (mEq/l)
Urea	13.3 mmol/l (BUN 80 mg/dl)
Creatinine	690 μmol/l (7.8 mg/dl)
Ca	1.7 mmol/l (6.8 mg/dl)
pH	7.22
PCO_2	45 mmHg (6 kPa)

213 Why are hydrofluoric burns different from other caustic burns and what is the proper treatment for these?

214 A 55-year-old patient who has undergone a colostomy, Hartman's procedure and colon resection for perforated diverticulitis is in the ICU. This patient has required intubation and ventilation for the development of multiple system organ failure in the postoperative period. The patient has evidence of organ dysfunction of the lungs, kidneys, and liver. When would you consider tracheostomy on this patient?

211–214: Answers

211 This patient has significant bullous emphysema. Tension pneumothorax should be ruled out. The giant bullae can trap air and cause mediastinal shift. Options include selective ventilation of the opposite side, increasing expiratory time, bronchodilator and, or, jet ventilation. Ultimately this patient underwent resection of the bulla (**211b**).

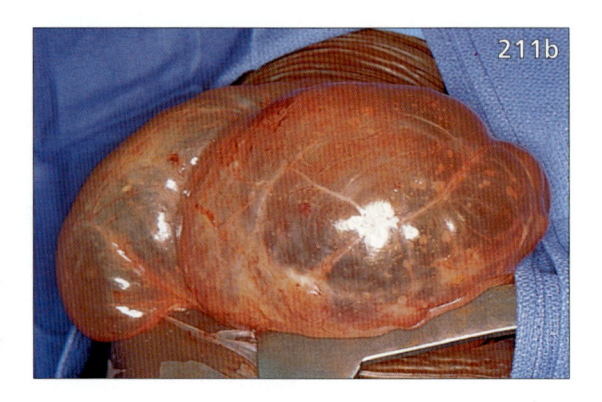

212 Hypermagnesemia (magnesium nitrate with renal failure) causes weakness, bradycardia, hyporeflexia and paralysis.

213 Hydrofluoric acid is used as a rust remover and a glass etching agent. It is tremendously caustic to biologic tissues, and will continue to cause liquefaction necrosis in tissues until neutralized with calcium solutions, which bind with the fluoride ion. Other caustic burns are not neutralized, but diluted with copious water irrigation. Typically, calcium gluconate solution is injected into the involved tissues. Optionally, a gel preparation can be made with calcium gluconate, which then is placed topically on the wounds.

214 Tracheostomy is generally considered in four situations: the prolonged need for mechanical ventilation with an artificial airway; the presence of airway obstruction or lack of access to the trachea above the larynx such as in trauma patients or patients with nasopharyngeal tumors; inadequate pulmonary toilet in handling pulmonary secretions, particularly with re-intubation; and inability to wean the patient from mechanical ventilation. There are two different philosophic approaches to tracheostomy. One is the performance of the tracheostomy at 24–48 hours if prolonged mechanical ventilation is anticipated. The other is continued use of an ET intubation which has a low pressure high volume cuff. It is not uncommon to proceed with this type of intubation for several weeks before the performance of tracheostomy. An intermediate approach is to use regular fiberoptic examination of the upper airway to assess the patient for laryngeal damage. Tracheostomy is performed when evidence of laryngeal damage is present. In neurologically impaired patients with limited chance for neurologic recovery, tracheostomy may be performed at an earlier time in order to wean the patient from the ventilator, but still protect the airway and provide access for secretion control.

215–217: Questions

HR 100/min
Systolic BP 120/80 mmHg
 (16.0/10.7 kPa)
Bilirubin 25.9 µmol/l (1.5 mg/dl)
Albumin 35 g/l (3.5g/dl)
Prothrombin time 11.5 seconds
 (normal)

215 This 45-year-old alcoholic male with a history of upper gastrointestinal bleeding presents with a second bleeding episode (**215**). He has a history of varices. These were treated with sclerotherapy 3 months previously. A nasogastric tube reveals the presence of blood within the stomach. The patient's laboratory results are shown. He has no ascites and no encephalopathy. Discuss the management of this patient.

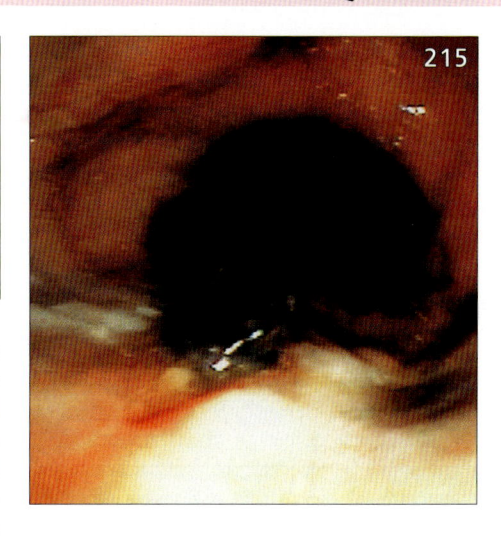

216 Which of the following cell types are essential for cutaneous wound repair?
A Polymorphonuclear leukocytes.
B Macrophages.
C T lymphocytes.
D Fibroblasts.
E Keratinocytes.
F Endothelial cells.

217 Status epilepticus is defined as:
A Continuous seizure activity >90 minutes.
B Continuous seizure activity >1 hour.
C Continuous seizure activity >30 minutes.
D Two or more sequential seizures with full recovery of consciousness between seizures.
E Seizures occurring for >30 minutes secondary to head trauma.

153

215–217: Answers

	Child's classification		
	A	B	C
Encephalopathy	None	Mild	Severe
Ascites	None	Slight	Moderate
Coagulopathy	Prothrombin time prolonged 1–4 sec	Prothrombin time prolonged 4–6 sec	Prothrombin time prolonged >6 sec
Bilirubin µmol/l (mg/dl)	<25.5 (<1.5)	25.5–51 (1.5–3.0)	>51 (>3.0)
Albumin g/l (g/dl)	>35 (3.5)	28–35 (2.8–3.5)	<28 (<2.8)

215 The initial management of variceal bleeding is that of any acute upper gastrointestinal bleed and includes the placement of a large IV catheters, transfusion, correction of coagulation defects, and early endoscopy. As many as 50% of patients with known varices will be bleeding from another site such as peptic ulcers or gastritis. Patients who have variceal bleeds that are severe can be managed initially with a Sengstaken–Blakemore tube. Subsequent management depends on the Child's classification (see table above).

Management of patients with A or B symptoms with a second bleed is usually surgical. Sclerotherapy either the first or second time is associated with up to a 50% rebleed rate with a mortality rate of approximately 30%. If the patient is not actively bleeding or is clinically stable, the best surgical option is selective distal splenorenal shunt as this is associated with a low incidence of encephalopathy. A complication of this is increased ascites. If the patient has a massive bleed and is not stable or has moderate ascites, a nonselective central shunt such as a portal cava shunt is recommended. This is associated with an increased rate of encephalopathy. The initial management of the patient with Child A or B symptomatology and first time bleed is controversial. Most centers would feel that sclerotherapy with repeat esophagoscopy and repeat sclerotherapy is the best initial management. Patients with Child C symptoms are most difficult. Medical options include Sengstaken–Blakemore tubes, vasopressin, and, or, somatostatin. Interventional procedures such as transhepatic intraparenchymal portosystemic shunting are associated with a 50% success rate and survival at 1 year. Some centers have advocated the Sugiura procedure with somatostatin postoperatively.

216 B, D, E, and F. Anti-sera studies deleting polymorphonuclear leukocytes, T cells and B cells did not cause a change in wound strength, but deletion of macrophages caused a profound loss of wound strength. Endothelial cells and fibroblasts are the main components of granulation tissue and keratinocytes provide epithelial coverage.

217 C. Status epilepticus is defined as more than 30 minutes of continuous seizure activity or two or more sequential seizures without full recovery of consciousness between seizures.

218–220: Questions

218 With regard to arterial catheters for monitoring, which of the following are true?
A In terms of reliability, smaller gauge catheters are more reliable.
B Radial artery catheters are as reliable as femoral lines in patients who are in shock or receiving high dose pressors.
C Patients can 'bleed to death' from radial arterial lines.
D The most common and potentially serious complication of intraarterial monitoring is pseudoaneurysm formation.

219 A 19-year-old male is struck by a motor vehicle while crossing the street. X-rays demonstrate nondisplaced right tibia and fibula fractures. Three hours after his arrival, he begins to complain of worsening pain in the leg. He is also noted to have intact pulses with pain to passive motion at the ankle. What is the next step in evaluating/treating this patient?
A Place ice bags on his leg and elevate to decrease swelling.
B Apply a plaster cast to immobilize the extremity.
C Obtain an electromyogram to rule out tibial nerve injury.
D Perform compartment pressure measures in all four compartments of the lower leg.

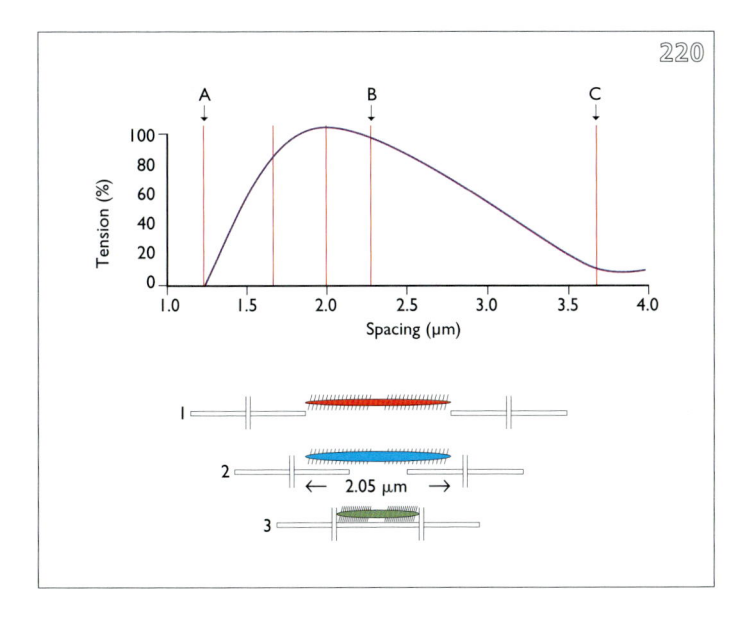

220 Fit the appropriate figures (1–3) illustrating the relationship of thick and thin filaments with the points on the graph (A–C) depicting developed tension (**220**).

218–220: Answers

218 A True: smaller catheters (20–24 gauge) allow more optimal dampening in a system, thus reducing systolic overshoot. In addition, larger catheters can occlude the smaller vessels resulting in distortion of the pulse signal.

B False: peripheral vasoconstriction under these circumstances, can lead to gross underestimation of central pressures. In the normotensive patient, the pressures are exaggerated in distal blood vessels.

C True: blood loss from an uncapped or disconnected 18 gauge arterial line can exceed 500 ml/min.

D False: the most common and potentially serious complication of intraarterial monitoring is inaccurate measurements that prompt major errors in treatment. Pseudoaneurysms usually occur approximately two weeks following removal of the catheter. This can be managed with duplex compression, but often requires surgical repair.

219 D. This patient has early signs of a lower leg compartment syndrome. Immediate measurement of his pressures is necessary to determine the need for fasciotomy. Advanced signs, such as weakness of the extensor hallucis longus muscle, decreased sensation over the first web space of the foot, or changes in the pulses at the ankle, require early fasciotomy. Long-term sequelae are foot drop, long-term parathesias, and ischemic (Volkmann's) contractures. Causes that increase compartment volume are postischemic swelling (such as following an arterial occlusion or injury), arterial hemorrhage, soft-tissue crush, fractures with swelling and bleeding, and postexertional swelling. Those that constrict the compartment include constrictive dressings or casts and burn injury with resultant eschar which limits swelling of the injured muscle. The compartment pressure is measured by using a direct measurement device such as needle and pressure transducer or the Stryker brand instrument. Normal compartment pressures range from 15–25 mmHg (2.0–3.3 kPa). When the compartment pressure reaches 30–40 mmHg (4.0–5.3 kPa), it is recommended that full fasciotomy of all involved compartments be performed.

220 The stroke work-end diastolic relationship (such as described by Frank–Starling curves) reflects the degree of cross bridging between the filaments. Figure 1/point C represents maximal 'stretch', so that the filaments cannot interact. This is the theoretical point at which there is 'falling off' of the Starling curve with excessive distension. Figure 2/point B represents the most efficient overlap of thick and thin filaments, and thus the greater generated tension. Figure 3/point A represents maximal crowding, with no more ability to contract.

221–224: Questions

221 A patient who is on cimetidine as prophylaxis against 'stress ulceration' begins to have a gastrointestinal bleed. A work-up ensues which includes upper gastrointestinal endoscopy with findings of erosive gastritis. The patient's platelet count, which in the past had been normal, now is found to be below $75 \times 10^9/l$ (75,000/mm^3). Despite multiple platelet transfusions, the patient continues to bleed and to run platelet counts at below $50-75 \times 10^9/l$ (50–75,000/mm^3). Would the appropriate next management step be to perform gastrectomy, or discontinue the cimetidine?

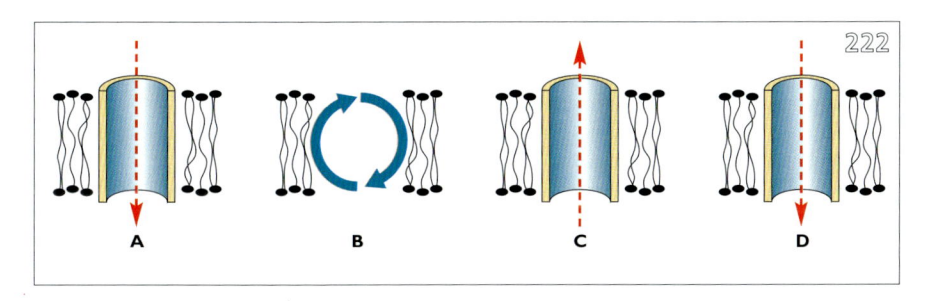

222 Identify the following passive channels of the cardiac plasma membrane (**222**). (Letters are on the intracellular side of the membrane.)

223 Which one of the blood gas profiles (A–D) in the table matches postoperative pneumonia in a patient with COPD.

	A	B	C	D
PaO$_2$ (mmHg (kPa))	105 (14.0)	108 (14.4)	36 (4.8)	50 (6.7)
SaO$_2$	100%	100%	58%	89%
PCO$_2$ (mmHg (kPa))	27 (3.6)	12 (1.6)	90 (12.0)	72 (9.6)
pH	7.55	7.05	7.25	7.46
HCO$_3^-$ (mmol/l, mEq/l)	23	5	38	50
BE	0	–30	+5	+20

224 i. Describe the relationship between bacterial translocation and multisystem organ failure seen in the critical care and postoperative patient setting.
ii. List factors that increase a patient's risk for developing this complication.
iii. Which nutritional intervention, total parenteral or enteral, is most frequently associated with this phenomenon?

221–224: Answers

221 Discontinue the cimetidine. Many drugs can cause thrombocytopenia. This can occur due to myelosuppression as from antineoplastic agents, or from immunologic mechanisms. Heparin is the most important cause of idiosyncratic drug induced thrombocytopenia, but a large number of other drugs, including the H_2 antagonist cimetidine, can lower platelet counts by producing a syndrome that mimics acute induced thrombocytopenia. The platelet count can begin to rise within a few days of discontinuing such agents.

222 A. The Na^+ channel is a fast channel that is controlled by a voltage dependent gate that is opened by depolarization to allow Na^+ entry. It is blocked by lidocaine, quinidine, and procainamide.
B. The Ca^{2+}/Na^+ exchange channel expels either Ca^{2+} or Na^+ depending upon intracellular concentrations of the ions.
C. The K^+ channel, allowing egress of K^+ from the cell, is opened by depolarization, and closed by repolarization.
D. The Ca^{2+} channel is controlled by two gate mechanisms. The outer gate is passive and voltage dependent. The inner gate opens to various degrees depending upon phosphorylation and is, therefore, mediated by cAMP. This slow channel is the target of the calcium channel blockers.

223 Blood gas profile C represents the postoperative pneumonia on a patient with COPD. This picture suggests acute respiratory acidosis or failure which is superimposed on chronic lung disease or chronic respiratory acidosis. In this particular patient, the severity of the ventilatory failure cannot be judged from the $PaCO_2$ alone. The pH is not severely acidemic and is not as great as the high PCO_2 would suggest. A small amount of supplemental oxygen may have a profound affect on arterial oxygenation and allow this patient to increase alveolar ventilation.

224 i. Bacterial translocation is a process by which bacteria migrate across the intestinal mucosal barrier to invade the liver, spleen, and mesenteric lymph nodes. In the gut-origin hypothesis of multisystem organ failure, translocated enteric bacteria and endotoxin travel to organs and tissues causing sepsis, macrophage cytokine secretion, neutrophil protease stimulation, oxidant production, proinflammatory endothelial cell promotion, and complement/coagulation system activation. (Evidence for this hypothesis has been demonstrated in laboratory experiments with animal models only.)
ii. Factors that increase risk or promote bacterial translocation include: mucosal damage from stress, starvation, radiation, and, or, chemotherapy, disruption of normal gastrointestinal flora, endotoxin, impaired immune function, hormonal factors associated with the lack of gastrointestinal stimulation, and nutrient specific deprivation.
iii. Parenteral nutrition has a hypoplastic effect on gastrointestinal mucosa, decreased mucosal enzyme activity, and decreased antral and circulating gastrin. The lack of enteral stimulation and presumed disruption of enteric flora increases the risk for bacterial translocation and subsequent sepsis.

225–227: Questions

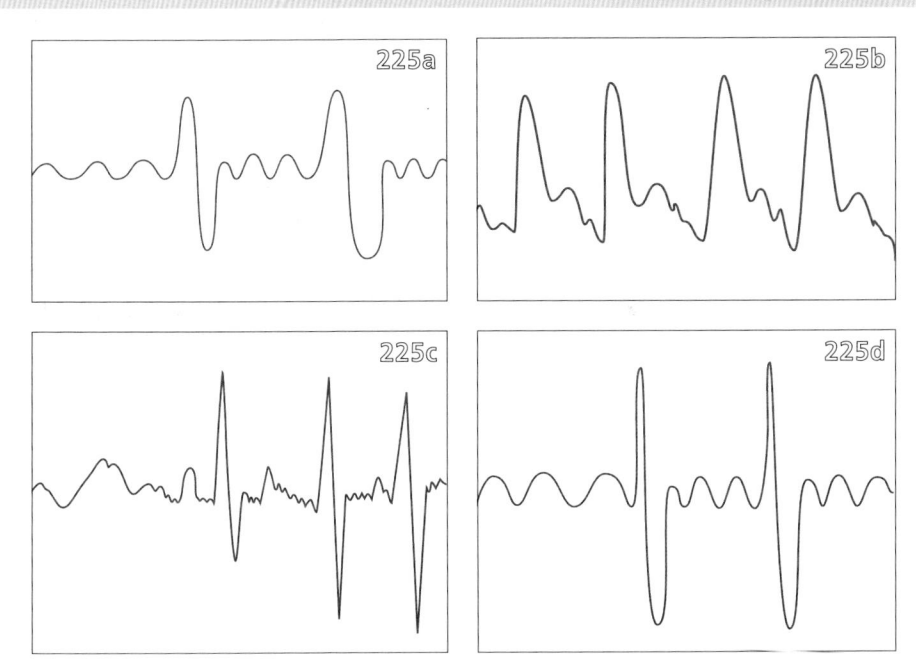

225 Diagnose the 'black board' representations of supraventricular dysrhythmias (225a–d).

226 What factors influence the speed of onset of inhalational agents?

227 Match the clinical condition with the change in $AVDO_2$ (normal 5% volume); either low (<5% volume) or high (>5% volume).
A Cardiomyopathy.
B Cirrhosis.
C Pheochromocytoma.
D Hypophosphatemia.
E Thyrotoxicosis.
F Thiamine deficiency.
G Pulmonary embolus.
H Arteriovenous fistula.
I Cocaine abuse.
J Temperature >39°C (102.2°F).

225–227: Answers

225 (**225a**) Atrial fibrillation with aberrency; (**225b**) atrial fibrillation; (**225c**) atrial fibrillation; (**225d**) supraventricular tachycardia with rate related ischemia. Atrial fibrillation implies chaotic ectopic rhythm from multiple ectopic sites and thus the baseline is very variable. Atrial flutter and supraventricular tachycardia represent re-entrant disturbances and, therefore, are more regular. A flutter usually has an atrial rate of 240–360/min but usually AV node blocks the ventricular rate at 1:2 or 1:3. The 'classic' ventricular rate is 150/min. Supraventricular tachycardia is similar except the re-entrant arrhythmia is transmitted completely via the AV node and the ventricular rate is 160–250/min.

226 General anesthesia with an inhalational agent is achieved when its concentrations in the CNS is sufficiently high to induce loss of consciousness. This is a result of a series of diffusion gradients between: (1) The inspired concentration and the tension in the alveolus. (2) The alveolus and the pulmonary capillary tension. (3) The pulmonary and cerebral capillary tension. (4) The cerebral blood tension and the CNS tissue concentration. As a result the speed of onset is mainly governed by the rapidity of the build-up of alveolar concentration. The alveolar concentration is determined by the property of the volatile agent and by patient factors. The rate of onset of an inhalational agent is dependent on its blood:gas solubility coefficient – the lower this is, the less soluble the agent is in blood and hence the more rapid will be the rise in alveolar concentration towards inspired tension. If, on the other hand, an agent is highly soluble in blood, it is extensively removed from the alveoli and the concentration there remains low. Onset of anesthesia is subsequently slow because the diffusion gradients are low. Patient factors which influence the speed of onset of anesthesia are pulmonary ventilation and cardiac output. The uptake of anesthetic is dependent on pulmonary ventilation and can thus be altered by changes in either ventilation or ventilation/perfusion ratios. Hyperventilation will increase the alveolar tension of inhalational agents and hence the diffusion gradients, so speeding the onset of anesthesia. Hypoventilation has the opposite effect. The functional residual capacity also affects the speed of onset. A larger functional residual capacity means that there is a larger 'buffer' between the alveolar gas and the inspired gas and slows the rate of rise of the alveolar concentration. Cardiac output can similarly alter the speed of induction by affecting the diffusion gradient between alveolus, pulmonary capillary blood and tissues. A reduced cardiac output, and hence pulmonary blood flow, will decrease the rate of removal of agent from the alveolus and produces a rapid rise in alveolar tension.

227 Low $AVDO_2$: B, E, F, H, J. High $AVDO_2$: A, C, D, G, I. A low $AVDO_2$ implies a hyperdynamic state usually with high cardiac output. These conditions include cirrhosis, thyrotoxicosis, thiamine deficiency (beriberi), arteriovenous fistula, hyperthermia, sepsis, and Paget's disease. A high $AVDO_2$ is seen with low cardiac output states including cardiogenic shock, cardiomyopathy, pheochromocytoma, the left ventricular failure caused by hypophosphatemia, pulmonary embolus, and toxic effects of drugs, such as arsenic and cocaine.

228–230: Questions

228 A 48-year-old male presents with a hematemesis of coffee-ground material. The examination of the stomach reveals erosive gastritis in the antrum and the lower esophagus shows the following findings (**228**). The patient has never bled before and he denies significant medical problems.
i. What is the finding?
ii. Name diseases associated with this condition.
iii. What would you do?

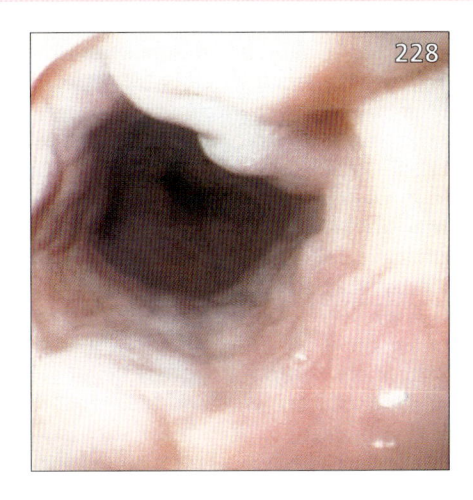

229 What is the creatine clearance in the following:
i. A 65-year-old male weighing 70 kg (154 lb). Serum creatine is 133 µmol/l (1.5 mg/dl).
ii. A 55-year-old female weighing 45 kg (99 lb). Serum creatine is 133 µmol/l (1.5 mg/dl).

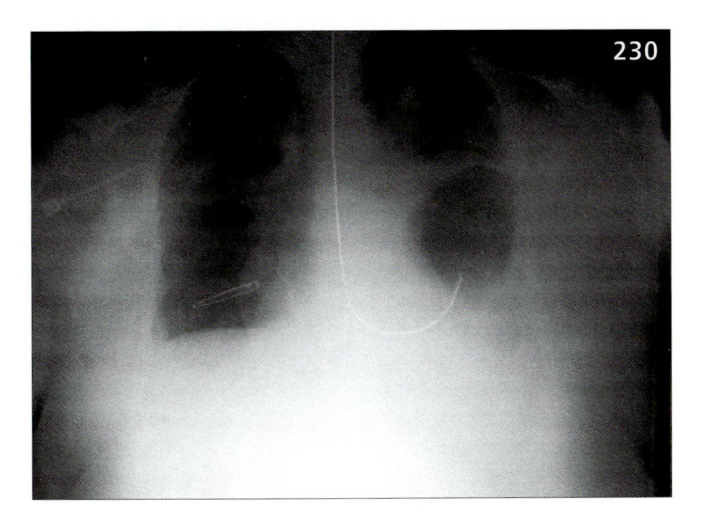

230 A 67-year-old female is being ventilated in your unit for pulmonary contusion and rib fractures following a motor vehicle accident. She is extubated and complains of chest pain. The X-ray is shown (**230**). What is your diagnosis and plan for therapy?

228–230: Answers

228 i. The picture shows esophageal varices. They do not demonstrate signs of recent hemorrhage (such as clots, red spots) and most likely the patient's gastritis is responsible for the bleeding. Esophageal varices are found in patients with portal hypertension. Most patients will have evidence for chronic liver disease on physical examination but in approximately 15% no clues are found.
ii. In western countries portal hypertension is most commonly caused by end-stage liver disease (cirrhosis) resulting from alcoholism, and hepatitis B and C. Other etiologies are metabolic liver diseases such as hemochromatosis, Wilson's disease, or autoimmune diseases such as primary biliary cirrhosis and chronic active hepatitis.

A whole different category are diseases that do not effect the liver parenchyma but rather cause portal hypertension due to thrombosis of the portal vein and splenic vein, or obstruction of the the inferior vena cava, hepatic vein, or venules.
iii. Only patients who have bled from their esophageal varices show a clear benefit from endoscopic therapy. Patients like the one presented may benefit from interventions such as alcohol abstinence (if alcoholism is the culprit) or beta-blocker therapy.

229 i. Creatine clearance in males can be estimated by the following:

$$\text{creatine clearance (ml/min)} = \frac{[(140-\text{age}) \text{ weight (kg)}]}{(72 \times \text{serum creatine})}$$

In this case creatine clearance = 48.6 ml/min.
ii. Creatine clearance in women can be estimated by multiplying the above by 0.85. In this case creatine clearance is approximately 30 ml/min.

230 This chest X-ray represents a ruptured diaphragm. The liver and the heart appear to buffer the right hemidiaphragm. Autopsy studies have demonstrated that the posterior aspect of the left diaphragm is somewhat weaker than the right diaphragm. Stomach, spleen, colon, and omentum can herniate through the opening into the chest causing acute respiratory distress. An upright chest X-ray is the best diagnostic test for diaphragmatic rupture. As in this case, the nasogastric tube may be seen above the level of the diaphragm. In the intubated, ventilated patient, the positive pressure in the thorax may prevent herniation of the intra-abdominal organs so that this injury may not be recognized until after the patient has been extubated. Small tears in the diaphragm are repaired with sutures. Large tears may require prosthetic material.

231–233: Questions

231 Two capnographs of two patients receiving CPR (**231a, b**). Which patient has a better prognosis?

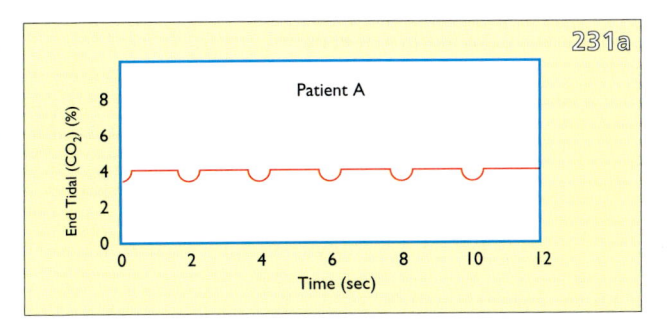

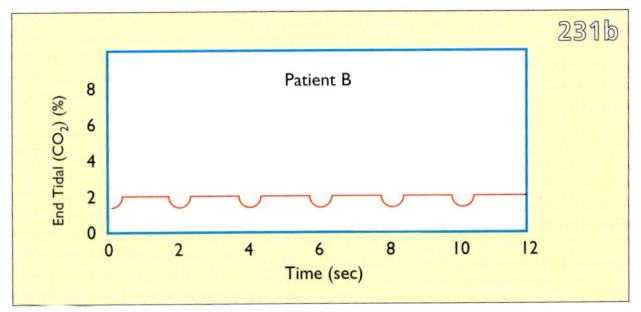

Patient A — End Tidal (CO$_2$) (%) vs Time (sec)

Patient B — End Tidal (CO$_2$) (%) vs Time (sec)

232 A patient with newly diagnosed nonsmall cell lung cancer remains in your unit because of failure to wean. A week ago, the oncologists gave him neoadjuvant chemotherapy. You are called because he is febrile with a temperature of 38.6°C (101.5°F). On examination, there is no obvious source for the temperature elevation. Review of laboratory data from that day reveals that the WBC is 1.2×10^9/l (1,200/mm^3) with 22% neutrophils. How do you respond?

233 Match the drug (A–D) with its hemodynamic effect (1–4).
A Esmolol.
B Nitroprusside.
C Dobutamine.
D Epinephrine.

Profile	Mean arterial pressure	Cardiac output	Systemic vascular resistance	Pulmonary capillary wedge pressure
1	None/increase	Increase	Decrease	Decrease
2	Decrease	Increase or decrease	Decrease	Decrease
3	Increase	Increase	Increase	Increase
4	Decrease	Decrease	None	None

231–233: Answers

231 Patient A. Without pulmonary blood flow, no CO_2 is delivered to the lungs, and consequently, none is exhaled. Effective chest compressions will resume circulation; as a result of returned blood flow to lungs, CO_2 will be exhaled, and the amounts can be measured by capnography. The amount of CO_2 returned to the lungs and subsequently exhaled, is proportional to the amount of pulmonary blood flow. Sharp increases in exhaled CO_2 during chest compresses are often predictive of a return to spontaneous circulation. Therefore, since patient A demonstrates greater amounts of exhaled CO_2 than patient B, patient A is expected to have a better prognosis.

232 An individual with a normal WBC count and distribution may be febrile without obvious source, and one may choose to observe without specific intervention. Febrile neutropenia, however, is an oncologic emergency. With few circulating granulocytes, the classic inflammatory signs may be absent, e.g. infected line exits may not appear red and chest X-rays may show no infiltrate. Infection in these circumstances, most often from the patient's own microbial flora, can include Gram-negative as well as Gram-positive organisms, and can progress from fever to death in a matter of hours. A single temperature of at least 38.3°C (100.9°F) orally in the absence of obvious environmental cause or a temperature that remains at least 38.0°C (100.4°F) orally for an 1 hour should be considered a fever. An absolute granulocyte count of 1,000 or less would constitute significant neutropenia. The response to febrile neutropenia should include a thorough physical examination with special attention to lungs, oral cavity, perineum, and skin. Laboratory studies should include chest X-ray and blood, sputum, and urine specimens for microbial culture. Empiric broad spectrum antibiotic coverage should begin immediately. One common approach is to combine an aminoglycoside with a beta-lactam penicillin. Other precautions applicable to the care of neutropenic patients include: placement in a private room, scrupulous adherence to hand washing, and avoidance of flowers, raw vegetables, and fruit without peelable skins. Failure of fever to remit after several days of appropriate antibacterial therapy is cause to broaden antibiotic spectrum further and ultimately to add antifungal coverage.

233 A and 4; B and 2; C and 1; D and 3. Esmolol is a short acting beta blocker. It has been used to control supraventricular tachycardia and postoperative hypertension. Severe hypotension is the most common adverse reaction. This drug causes a decrease in arterial BP, a decrease in the cardiac output and HR, with no effect on either systemic vascular resistance or pulmonary capillary wedge pressure. Nitroprusside is both an arterial and venovasodilator. It is used as an antihypertensive agent. Nitroprusside decreases mean arterial pressure, decreases systemic vascular resistance and pulmonary capillary wedge pressure, and may either increase or decrease cardiac output. Dobutamine is a positive inotropic, chronotropic, and vasodilating agent. It is used primarily to improve myocardial contractility and stroke volume. It has little effect or may slightly increase mean arterial pressure, increase cardiac output, decreases systemic vascular resistance, and decreases pulmonary capillary wedge pressure. Epinephrine is a naturally occurring catecholamine which is a potent vasoconstrictor. Epinephrine increases mean arterial pressure, cardiac output, systemic vascular resistance, and pulmonary capillary wedge pressure.

234–236: Questions

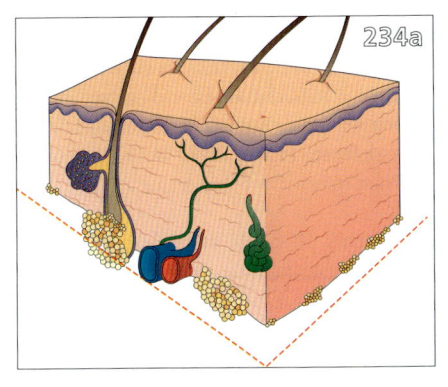

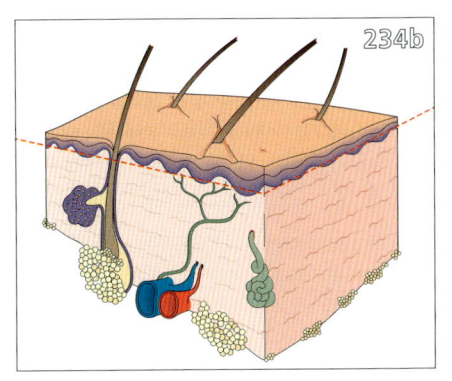

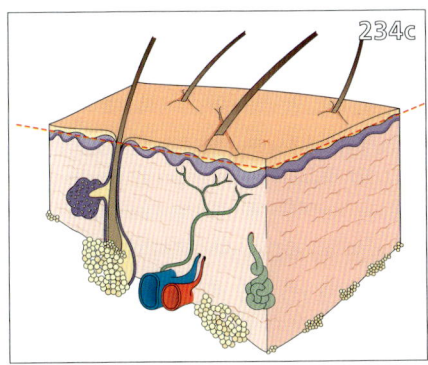

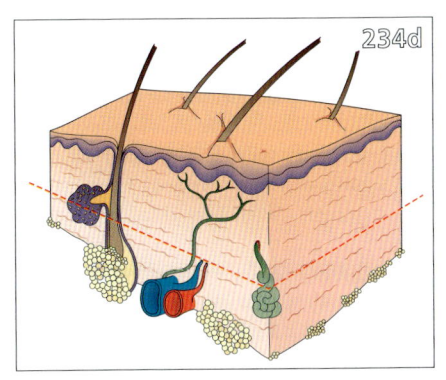

234 Above are four different depths of burns indicated by the red line (**234a–d**). Assign a degree of severity to each.

235 Initial treatment of anaphylactic shock is:
A Benadryl.
B Epinephrine (adrenaline).
C Dopamine.
D Norepinephrine (noradrenaline).
E Corticosteriods.

236 A patient with acute pancreatitis is admitted to the ICU with tachypnea, a BP of 100 mmHg (13.3 kPa), HR of 130/min, and an urine output of 20 ml/hr.
i. How would you resuscitate this patient?
ii. What other diagnostic studies would you consider in this patient after resuscitation?

234–236: Answers

234 Figure **234a** is a third degree burn, where all elements of the skin including 'appendages' (sweat glands and hair follicles) are burned, thereby resulting in no capability of self-healing. Figure **234b** demonstrates a superficial second degree burn, with the uppermost elements of the dermis involved as well. Figure **234c** is a superficial first degree burn, confined wholly to the epidermal layer. Figure **234d** demonstrates a deep second degree burn, with involvement of the vast majority of the dermis.

235 B. Epinephrine is the drug of choice since it treats all of the major physiological sequelae of acute anaphylaxis. It will bronchodilate and increase vascular peripheral resistance (afterload) supporting BP. Other drugs can be used for secondary management. *They are not a substitute for epinephrine (adrenaline)*. These include albuterol or aminophylline for bronchospasm. Hydrocortisone (500 mg) as anti-inflammatory therapy and a histamine (H_1) antagonist, such as chlorpheniramine (20 mg), are frequently recommended to treat the immune response cascade. Dopamine and norepinephrine (noradrenaline) are indicated for hypotension refractory to epinephrine and fluids.

236 i. Patients with pancreatitis have tremendous fluid losses. The pancreatitis acts like a burn of the peritoneal cavity and causes tremendous third spacing of fluids in the abdomen. With this third spacing of fluids, hypovolemia can occur. The other aspect of pancreatic disease is the hemorrhagic component of pancreatitis. Hemoglobin must, therefore, be checked and monitored. This patient should be given aggressive fluid resuscitation similar to that given to a trauma patient. BP, HR, and urine output can be used as guides to fluid resuscitation, as can invasive central venous lines or pulmonary artery catheters. Patients with pancreatitis also develop respiratory failure with either pleural effusion or ARDS. Blood gas monitoring and serial chest radiographs are important. While monitoring BP and urine output, 2 l of crystalloid can be rapidly infused. If there is no effect from the fluid resuscitation, hemodynamic monitoring should be instituted. Fluid resuscitation can be guided by either the rise in wedge pressure or the rise in CVP or alternatively, the change in cardiac output.

ii. There are three surgically correctable causes of pancreatitis. One is trauma where you can have either pancreatitis or actual pancreatic transection. The second is biliary tract disease and the third is a penetrating ulcer. A clinical history from the patient or the family of any pre-existing conditions is important: medications, including thiazide diuretics and corticosteroids, alcohol abuse or hyperglycemia. Diagnostic studies include an ultrasound of the right upper quadrant to evaluate the presence of biliary tract disease, evaluation for ulcer disease (endoscopy), and a CT scan of the abdomen to evaluate the pancreas for pancreatic necrosis and abscess formation. Surgical intervention in patients with acute pancreatitis is indicated with hemorrhagic pancreatitis, pancreatic necrosis, and pancreatic abscess formation.

237–239: Questions

237 A 59-year-old male (weighing 55 kg/121 lb) underwent surgical resection for bowel perforation. He has no significant past medical history. His family history is negative for diabetes. He was started on central total parenteral nutrition postoperatively using dextrose and amino acid to provide a total of 2,700 kcal. His blood-work results the next morning are shown.

Na+ 139 mmol/l (mEq/l)
K+ 4.3 mmol/l (mEq/l)
Cl− 100 mmol/l (mEq/l)
HCO_3^- 25 mmol/l (mEq/l)
Glucose 17.8 mmol/l (321 mg/dl)

i. What metabolic complication of total parenteral nutrition is the patient experiencing?
ii. What are potential sequelae of this metabolic complication?
iii. What are the options for management of this complication?

238 A patient has been on long-term parenteral nutrition. She develops signs of sepsis and her left upper extremity is noted to be swollen. Her chest X-ray is shown (**238**). Blood cultures drawn through the central line and peripherally are both positive for *Enterobacter* species. An echocardiogram is performed which demonstrates a clot along the catheter tip with subclavian vein thrombosis. Discuss the management of line sepsis.

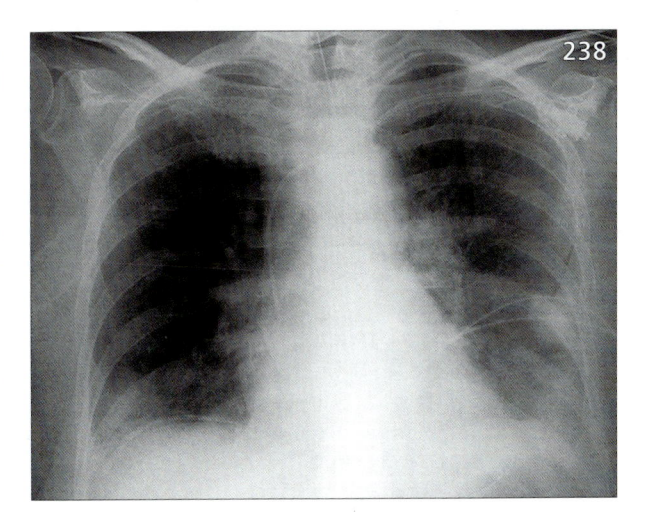

239 Which of the following antidotes (A–E) can be considered for the corresponding toxic agents (1–5)?

A N-acetylcystein.
B Physostigmine.
C Thiosulfate.
D Ethanol.
E Atropine.

1 Cyanide.
2 Organic phosphates.
3 Methanol.
4 Anticholinergics.
5 Acetaminophen.

237–239: Answers

237 i. The patient is experiencing hyperglycemia secondary to total parenteral nutrition. Patients who are under medical/surgical stress have increased counter-regulatory hormones (i.e. epinephrine (adrenaline), cortisol, and glucagon) which increases hepatic gluconeogenesis and decreases peripheral muscle uptake of glucose. This 'stress response' leads to insulin resistance and subsequent hyperglycemia.
ii. Elevated blood glucose has been associated with immunosuppressive effects, such as decreased chemotaxis/phagocytosis. Studies have substantiated that hyperglycemia is associated with an increased risk of infections. Other complications include fluid/electrolyte abnormalities, and hyperglycemic, hyperosmotic, and nonketotic coma.
iii. Total parenteral nutrition-induced hyperglycemia may be managed in several ways. These include: addition of insulin to the total parenteral nutrition solution itself; insulin administration peripherally using a 'sliding-scale' based on finger-stick glucose monitoring; the use of lipid as a calorie source; or the lowering of total calorie provisions. The selection of strategy should be changed in accordance with the individual patient's clinical presentation.

238 Prevention of line sepsis requires aseptic placement techniques and frequent (every 24–48 hours) dressing changes with antibiotic ointment and occlusive dressings. The site easiest to keep 'clean' is the infraclavicular subclavian access. The incidence of line sepsis has been linked to the number of ports (3–5% per port), the rate of usage of the port, and the length of time the line is in place. Most centers advocate 'reguidewiring' the line periodically (between 2–7 days). The diagnosis of line sepsis is often one of exclusion (this patient, for example, was 4 days postoperative from a small bowel resection). However, purulent drainage, erythema, and, or, extremity swelling should suggest the diagnosis. If the blood culture is positive, but all other potential sources are negative, the line should be cultured. If there is only suspicion of line sepsis, the line can be 're-wired' and the intracutaneous portion (which has a higher detection rate than the tip) sent for culture. Line sepsis is confirmed if more than 15 colonies grow. If the catheter and peripheral blood cultures are negative, but the blood drawn through the catheter is positive, line sepsis is assumed. Treatment can include intravenous antibiotics through the new line. A more definitive method is to remove the line, treat with appropriate antibiotics for 7 days, and place a new catheter through a separate site either after fever has abated or after 24–48 hours of antibiotics. In this case there is evidence of line sepsis, as well as infected thrombosis of the subclavian, and along the catheter. In addition, there are peripheral 'infarcts' in the chest X-ray, consistent with emboli. This patient needs at a minimum to have the line removed, and be treated with heparin for septic pulmonary emboli. Some patients will develop a fixed infected thrombus of the atrium and, or, cardiac valves, possibly requiring surgery to remove/debride all infected tissue.

239 A and 5.
B and 4.
C and 1.
D and 3.
E and 2.

240–242: Questions

240 The CT scans (**240a–c**) are obtained from an 11-year-old male after a motor vehicle accident. He was the rear seat passenger. He has a BP of 140/80 mmHg (18.7/10.7 kPa), HR of 120/min, and RR of 18/min. What should be done next?

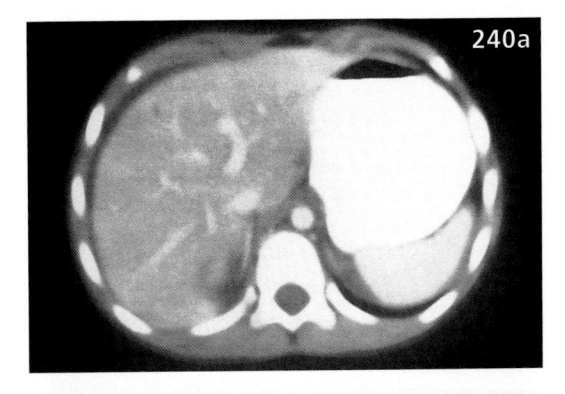

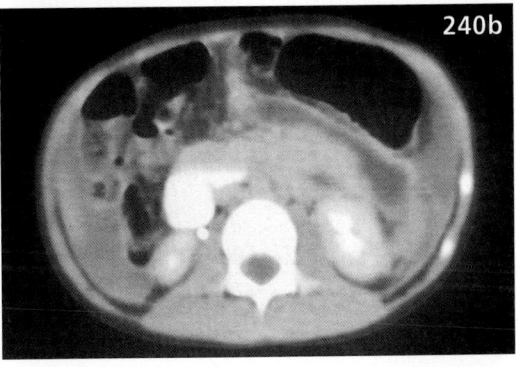

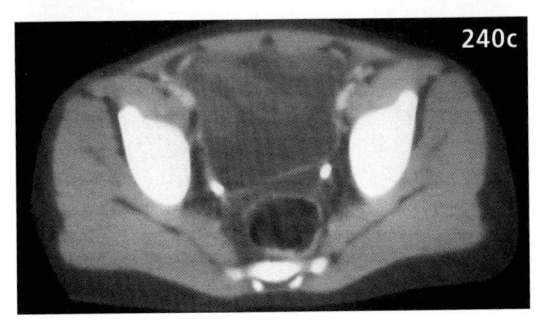

241 Discuss the role of aspirin and thrombolytic therapy in the acute management of myocardial infarction.

242 Your patient has a confirmatory test demonstrating colon ischemia following abdominal aortic aneurysm repair. Which patients are at greatest risk for this complication? How commonly does it occur? What should be done for these patients?

240–242: Answers

240 This CT scan shows fluid around the liver and in the pelvis. There is no parenchymal damage to the liver, spleen or kidneys. In the clinical circumstance of trauma, fluid surrounding these solid organs must be presumed to come from a bowel injury or intra-abdominal rupture of the bladder. However, the bladder in this case is intact. Blunt injury to the small bowel is more common than blunt injury either to the duodenum or the colon. Approximately 80% of small bowel injuries occur from the ligament of Treitz to the terminal ileum. The cause of small bowel injury is either crushing the small bowel against the vertebral column or by shearing and tearing. Under rare circumstances, a sudden increase in intraluminal pressure of the small bowel can cause perforation. Trauma to the small bowel is the third most common intra-abdominal injury following blunt trauma after spleen and liver. This patient should be prepared for operation with fluid resuscitation and antibiotics. The small bowel can be completely transected in one or more places or become ischemic from mesenteric disruption. Contusions of the small bowel can also occur. These areas may undergo subsequent necrosis and perforation after a relatively asymptomatic period. Small perforations of the bowel are repaired. Larger injuries and mesenteric injuries may require small bowel resection with anastomosis. Contusions are inverted or if extensive, resected.

241 There is a benefit to thrombolytic therapy if it is administered within 12 hours of the onset of symptoms of myocardial infarction, preferably within 90 minutes. Thrombolytic therapy and aspirin (including possibly prehospital thrombolytic therapy) should be considered in patients with ECG evidence of acute ischemia (ST elevation and, or, bundle branch block) and clinical signs and symptoms. Thrombolytic therapy should not be given in patients whose ECGs remain normal or exhibit only T-wave changes or ST depression (as these patients experience the risk of therapy but do not appear to have the same risk as a fully evolving myocardial infarction). Thrombolytic therapy is usually excluded for infarction established for more than 12 hours unless there is evidence of ongoing ischemia that meets criteria for thrombolysis. Thrombolysis is contraindicated in the following circumstances: stroke; recent major surgery (in the past 3 weeks); gastrointestinal intestinal bleeding within 1 month; a known bleeding disorder; aneurysm. Relative contraindications include: transient ischemia shock within 6 months; coumarin therapy; pregnancy; noncompressible venopunctures; traumatic resuscitation; refractory hypertension with systolic BP of more than 180 mmHg (24.0 kPa); recent retinal surgery.

242 The report incidence of intestinal ischemia following abdominal aortic aneurysm repair is from 0.2–10%. When prospectively studied by performing colonoscopy on all abdominal aortic aneurysm patients, an incidence of 6% was found. Risk factors for ischemia include: operation for aneurysm rather than occlusive disease, ruptured abdominal aortic aneurysm, prior colon resection, 'redo' grafting of the aorta, and suprarenal aortic clamping. Mucosal ischemia is treated conservatively with bowel rest, antibiotics and total parenteral nutrition. Transmural necrosis requires resection of the entire left colon including distal transverse colon and rectal closure below the peritoneal reflection. Colostomy and Hartmann's procedure are generally performed. Mortality for this complication ranges from 50–80%.

243–246: Questions

243 Correlate the areas of infarction in the figure (**243, A–C**) with the vessel distribution involved and ECG changes.

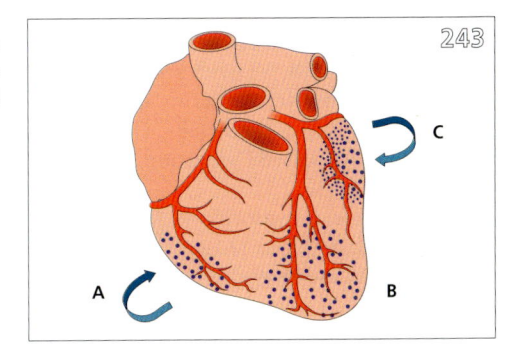

244 A patient with a severe hydrochloric acid injury of the upper gastrointestinal tract will require which of the following?
A A gastrostomy alone if there is gastric necrosis.
B Esophagectomy alone with immediate or delayed reconstruction by the stomach.
C Laparotomy. The main indication for this is abdominal tenderness.
D Esophagogastrectomy is required if gastric necrosis is found.

245 You are called to see a patient in the ICU because of a sudden desaturation according to his pulse oximeter. You know that he has bilateral tube thoracostomies, is intubated, ventilated, and that he is restrained because of agitation. His supine chest X-ray is shown (**245**). What is your diagnosis?

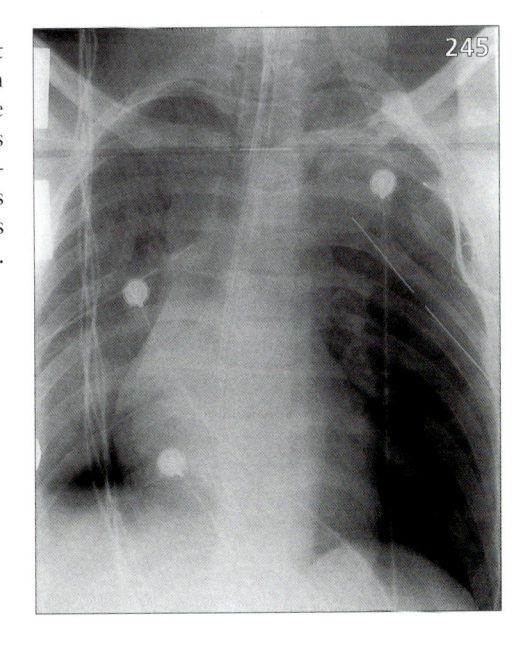

246 How does CT grading correlate with the risk of vasospasm in subarachnoid hemorrhage?

243–246: Answers

243 A. Inferior myocardial infarction; right coronary artery/patent ductus arteriosus; ST elevation in II, III, VF with reciprocal depression in V1–3. B. Anterior/apical myocardial infarction; left anterior descending artery/diagonals; ST elevation V1–3 (anteroseptal) V3–5 (anterior). C. Anterolateral myocardial infarction; circumflex/obtuse marginals; ST elevation V4–6, I, and VL.

244 E. A review of hydrochloric acid injuries shows that acid itself is more injurious to the stomach than the esophagus. However, patients who require gastric resection often have associated esophageal injury which causes either stenosis or further problems and are best treated by esophagogastrectomy. Abdominal tenderness for the laparotomy is a poor sign and a much better indication of severe gastric necrosis is CNS abnormalities.

245 Although difficult to call on supine chest films, this patient has a right pneumothorax. These are seen much more easily in an upright film, which was not available because of this patient's agitation and restrained state. The usual upright portable film in the ICU is relatively sensitive for pneumothoraces, showing the collection of air at the apices or laterally. If the lung markings are followed to the chest wall, a white line can be seen. This line is the interface between the lung and the pneumothorax. Findings are more subtle in the supine patient. Air collects anteriorly and is difficult to see, as it overlies normal lung tissue in this view. The air can collect along the medial heart border or along the diaphragm in these cases. Supine films may show nothing at all, they may show a medial dark area or a 'sulcus sign' meaning deepening of the lateral sulcus. With this clinical history, most likely causes are equipment failure. An agitated patient can easily dislodge any and all of their various tubes and lines. A comprehensive check of the tubing and all attachments from wall suction to tube entrance into the chest should be undertaken. In an emergent situation with an unstable picture, needle thoracostomy followed by definitive tube thoracostomy can also be used.

246 A CT grade by Fischer scale, if obtained within a few days, is useful in that patients with grade 3 are at increased risk for vasospasm. *Grade 1*: no subarachnoid hemorrhage. *Grade 2*: subarachnoid hemorrhage <1 mm. *Grade 3*: subarachnoid hemorrhage >1 mm. *Grade 4*: intracerebral or intraventricular subarachnoid hemorrhage bleed with no or thin (<1 mm) subarachnoid hemorrhage.

247–249: Questions

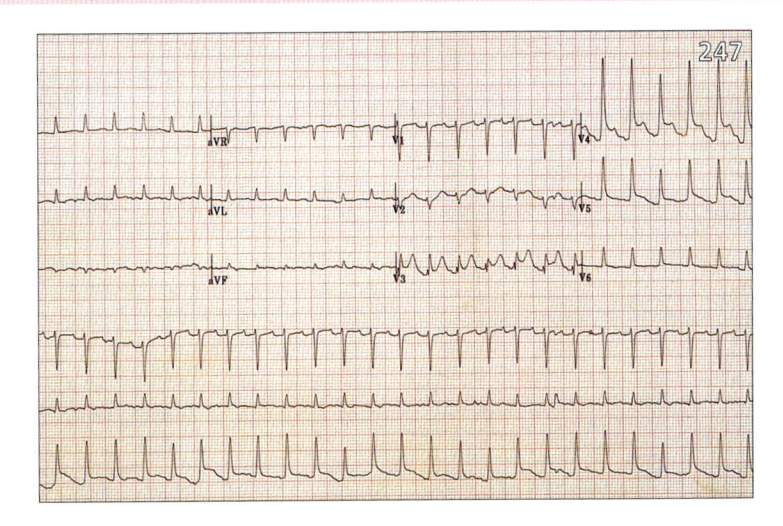

247 An ECG is undertaken intraoperatively on your newest admission to the ICU. This ECG was obtained soon after placement of an aortic cross clamp during emergency surgery for a ruptured abdominal aortic aneurysm (247). What does this show? Why did this happen?

248 A 65-year-old male with known coronary artery disease and CHF is being treated in the ICU for septic shock secondary to pneumonia. The patient is placed on a norepinephrine (noradrenaline) drip to maintain his mean arterial pressure above 70 mmHg (9.3 kPa). The patient develops diarrhea which is Guaiac positive. Physical examination reveals a distended, diffusely tender abdomen but without peritoneal signs. Blood work demonstrates lactic acidosis. Which of the following is the most likely diagnosis?
A Small bowel obstruction.
B Lower gastrointestinal bleeding most likely secondary to colonic angiodysplasia.
C Lower gastrointestinal bleeding of diverticular origin.
D Mesenteric ischemia.
E Ogilvie's syndrome.

249 A 44-year-old patient who was involved in a motor vehicle accident is admitted to the ICU after evacuation of a subdural hematoma. Blood loss was replaced appropriately during the operation. The patient's vital signs were stable during the surgical procedure and in the immediate postoperative period. There has been a 4 g drop in hemoglobin over the first 4 hours in the ICU. How would you evaluate this patient?

247–249: Answers

247 This patient has ST-T changes consistent with myocardial infarction. Cardiac ischemia is often the result of acute aortic occlusion which causes a significant sudden rise in afterload. Surgery for rupture generally involves supraceliac clamping because of the need for rapid access to the aorta. While infrarenal clamping is less hemodynamically significant, suprarenal clamping is severe. The renal vessels generally account for 22% of the cardiac output and the superior mesenteric artery and celiac trunk account for another 27%. Thus, the application of the supraceliac clamp puts the patient at significant cardiac risk in a setting where the anesthesiologist has little time to prepare the patient hemodynamically before this significant insult.

248 D. This patient probably has nonocclusive mesenteric ischemia resulting from low flow in the mesenteric circulation. It is secondary to the hypoperfusion related to his septic shock and underlying CHF and the direct vasospastic effect of the norepinephrine (noradrenaline) on the mesenteric arterial circulation. The norepinephrine drip should be stopped and the patient should be aggressively resuscitated with crystalloid and, or, colloids as indicated to optimize his cardiac output. If the patient does not respond to the above, an angiogram with selective catheterization of the superior mesenteric artery should be obtained to exclude acute occlusion and to selectively infuse vasodilators (e.g. papaverine) if extensive spasm or alternating spasm and dilation of the superior mesenteric artery branches, with impaired filling of the intramural bowel vessels, is seen. If the patient's condition deteriorates further and he develops peritoneal findings or free air on plain abdominal X-ray, he should undergo exploratory celiotomy. The clearly infarcted segments of bowel are resected, and the remaining bowel is left in the abdomen without anastomosis. The patient is returned to the ICU for further optimization of his cardiovascular status and sepsis. The patient should return to the operating room for a second-look procedure within the next 24 hours at which time the viability of the remaining bowel is reassessed and enteric continuity is reestablished.

249 A careful head-to-toe physical examination must be carried out. Examination of the chest for any evidence of hemothorax should be performed. A chest radiograph may be helpful. The pelvis and extremities must be carefully examined for any fracture site. If a pelvic radiograph is not already obtained, it should assist in evaluation of hidden blood loss. Bleeding into the abdomen can be assessed by a variety of techniques including diagnostic peritoneal lavage. A trauma echo should include views of the liver, spleen, and suprapubic areas as well as show fluid. A CT scan of the abdomen can be considered in stable patients. A diagnostic laparoscopy can be performed. If hypotension occurs in this scenario, an exploratory laparotomy is advised, providing there is a normal chest X-ray, no extremity fractures, and a normal pelvic X-ray.

250–253: Questions

250 Using the illustration of an action potential of a myocardial cell (**250**):
i. What do the 'phases' (0–4) represent?
ii. Which phase correlates with the QRS complex on the ECG?

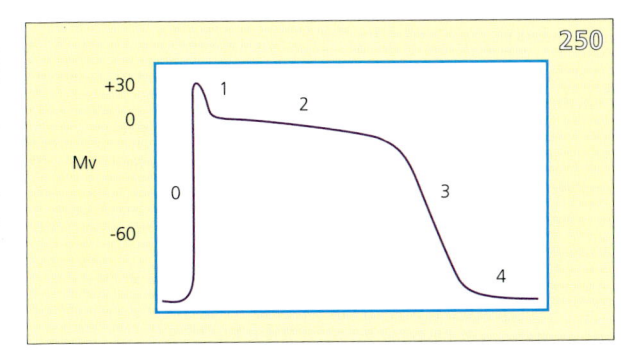

251 What are the airway considerations in this patient (**251**) who needs to undergo a thoracotomy for a lung abscess?

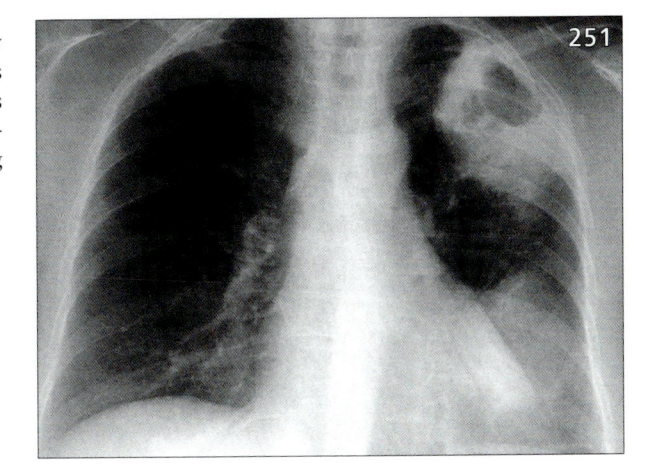

252 A 19-year-old male presents to the emergency department with a gunshot wound to the abdomen. His vital signs are HR 120/min, BP 96/66 mmHg (12.8/8.8 kPa), and RR 22/min. Two large bore antecubital IV catheters are placed and he receives 1 l of lactated Ringer's solution. His vital signs after fluid are HR 102/min, BP 115/76 mmHg (15.3/10.1 kPa), and RR 22/min. A right subclavian pulmonary artery catheter is inserted and a Resiscath monitoring device which measures SVO_2 is placed. His SVO_2 is 50%. Is this patient still in shock?

253 What is the management of bronchospasm in a ventilated patient?

250–253: Answers

250 i. Phase 0 represents depolarization, with opening of the fast Na$^+$ and K$^+$ channels. Closure of the Na$^+$ channels initiates a return to towards 0, initiating repolarization (phase 1). During phase 2, Ca^{2+} enters through slow channels. During phase, 3 K$^+$ efflux returns the membrane potential back to –90 mV, but the normal ionic gradient is not achieved until phase 4, when the active sodium-potassium pump exchanges Na$^+$ for K$^+$.
ii. Phase 0 correlates with the QRS complex on an ECG. Phase 2 correlates with the ST segment of the ECG.

251 This patient is at risk of the rupture of the abscess into the bronchi, with subsequent widespread tracheobronchial contamination. Options include the use of endobronchial blockers and advancing a single lumen tube into the opposite mainstem bronchus. However, the use of a double lumen tube is the more usual practice. Occasionally, patients with a lung abscess can be operated on in the prone position to keep the infected areas dependent.

252 Yes. Monitoring of vital signs (HR and BP) is standard in the resuscitation of shock patients. When these variables return to normal the assumption is that tissue oxygenation is adequate. However, numerous studies have revealed that despite normal vital signs there may be diminished tissue oxygenation. One study found that 50% of patients resuscitated from shock to normal vital signs had an abnormally low SVO$_2$ which correlated with the presence of lactic acidosis suggesting oxygen debt. Normal SVO$_2$ in this patient should be between 65–75%. The low SVO$_2$ indicates that his tissue beds are extracting oxygen at an abnormally high rate. Hypovolemic shock models show SVO$_2$ to be a more sensitive indicator of significant blood loss despite normal vital signs.

253 Simple bronchospasm should be treated by checking ET tube position and correcting if required, then by giving a beta$_2$ adenoreceptor agonist such as albuterol. This can be given directly by instilling 2.5–5 mg of nebulizer solution with some sterile saline down the ET tube and manually ventilating the lungs. This may prove difficult in the presence of significant airways obstruction and it often must be given intravenously in a dose of 3–4 mg/kg (approximately 200–300 mg for the average adult). This usually improves wheeze and oxygen saturation, but often causes significant tachycardia. Second line therapy includes aminophylline (6 mg/kg IV slowly over 20 minutes; average adult dose 400–600 mg), epinephrine (2 mg/kg IV boluses; average adult bolus 100 mg).

254–256: Questions

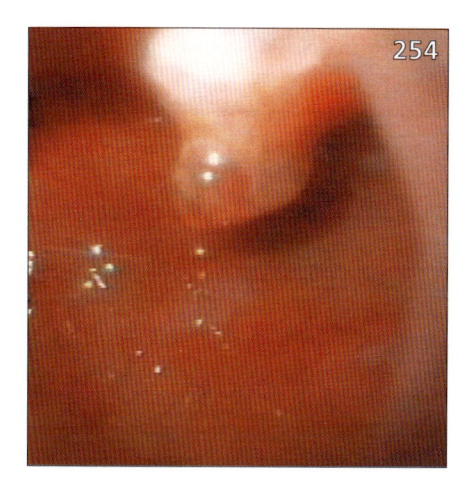

254 A 65-year-old male with atrial fibrillation on chronic anticoagulation is admitted to the hospital with a 2-week history of melena and fatigue. He complains of midepigastric pain, dizziness, and lightheadedness. There is no nausea, emesis, or hematemesis. An endoscopy is performed (**254**).
i. What is the finding?
ii. Which factors have been associated with increased morbidity and mortality in patients with gastrointestinal bleeding?
iii. What treatment modalities can be offered to this patient?

255 A 40-year-old female with C6 quadriplegia had a tracheostomy performed four weeks ago and is currently in the ICU being treated for respiratory failure secondary to a pneumonia. For the past 24 hours the nurse has occasionally noticed bloody aspirates on suctioning the patient's tracheostomy tube. You are at the bedside examining the patient when suddenly you notice bright red blood slowly oozing out from around the tracheostomy tube. You deflate the tube cuff and now the bleeding becomes massive. What should you do?
A Get a disseminated intravascular coagulation (DIC) profile and order 2 units of fresh frozen plasma.
B E-aminocaproic acid may be helpful in achieving local hemostasis.
C Reinflate the tube and let the surgeons know they will have to perform an emergency sternotomy in the operating room.
D Reinflate the tube and hold pressure over the tracheostomy incision, in situations like that the bleeding usually stops by this simple maneuver.

256 What is the risk of line sepsis from arterial monitoring lines?

254–256: Answers

254 i. This is a gastric ulcer with a visible vessel found in the antrum of the stomach. Ulcers are classified according to the endoscopic findings after Forrest: Ia spurting vessel, Ib nonspurting active bleeding, IIa visible vessel, IIb nonbleeding ulcer with a clot, IIc ulcer with hematin covered base, and III clean ulcer ground.
ii. The following factors have been associated with adverse outcomes from a gastrointestinal bleeding: advanced age, presence of comorbid conditions, coagulopathy, onset of bleeding while admitted to the hospital, magnitude of the bleeding (presence of shock), variceal bleeding compared to a nonvariceal bleeding, and certain endoscopic features (according to Forrest classification).
iii. Endoscopic hemostasis is generally recommended for patients with Forrest Ia, Ib, IIa, and subsets of patients with IIb. Techniques currently used include injection therapy with epinephrine (adrenaline), heater probe, and thermocoagulation, as well as the endoscopic clipping technique (used in European centers). The treatment for patients who failed endoscopic therapy remains largely surgical but in individual patients a repeat trial can be considered.

255 C. The patient has a tracheoinnominate fistula which manifested itself by intermittent herald bleeding with suctioning of the tracheostomy tube for the past 24 hours. The diagnosis was confirmed when the bleeding became massive upon deflation of the tracheostomy tube balloon. Tracheoinnominate fistula is a rare but very serious complication of tracheostomy. It usually occurs when the tracheostomy is performed too low – below the fourth tracheal ring. Direct erosion of the lower edge of the tube into the adjacent anteriorly coursing innominate artery is the usual etiology of the fistula. Control of the bleeding should be attempted by overinflation of the tracheostomy tube cuff against the innominate artery. If this fails the pretracheal space should be carefully dissected and a finger inserted to compress the bleeding artery against the posterior aspect of the sternum while the patient is transferred to the operating room. Alternatively, re-unlabeling in a no. 6 FRETT and holding pressure by a finger placed into the trachea itself can be done. Immediate median sternotomy should then be done to control the innominate artery and its branches. The involved portion of the innominate should then be resected and the proximal and distal ends should be oversewn. Reconstruction of the innominate artery in this situation is ill-advised because of the risks of infection and recurrent bleeding. The incidence of adverse neurologic sequelae from interruption of the innominate artery is relatively low, particularly in young patients.

256 Local infection and catheter colonization occur 10–15%. This risk is higher with cut down techniques. Systemic sepsis is uncommon (0.2–5%), and the incidence is related to the duration of catheter use and contamination of the infiltrate. Infection rates are much lower than seen with central venous and pulmonary artery catheters.

257, 258: Questions

257 A 45-year-old male with injuries sustained in a motor vehicle accident presents to the emergency room comatose with a systolic arterial BP of 90 mmHg (12.0 kPa), HR of 110/min, and a RR of 33/min. Soon after intubation and ventilation, he deteriorates with lack of palpable pulses. You:
A Immediately open the chest and perform open cardiac massage.
B Transfuse blood.
C Auscultate the chest.
D Do a diagnostic peritoneal lavage.
E Reintubate the patient.

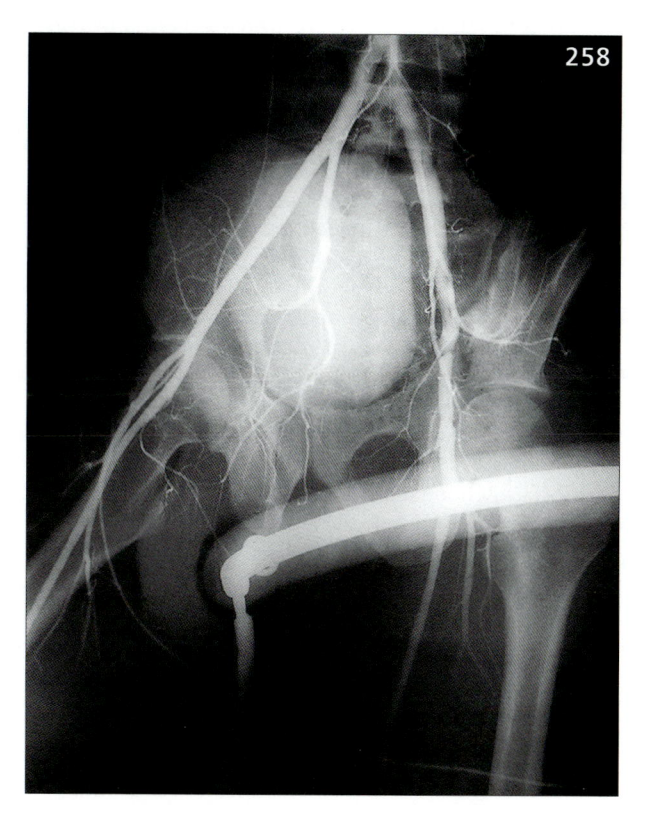

258 A 60-year-old restrained male was involved in a head-on motor vehicle accident. He presented with decreased pulses which prompted the angiogram shown (**258**). The next step in the management is:
A Laparotomy.
B Groin incision with crossover femoro–femoral bypass.
C Observation.
D Heparin.

257, 258: Answers

257 C. Causes for arrest include ET malposition, increased intrathoracic pressure, and metabolic problems. During intubation visualization of the ET tube passing through the cords is imperative for correct placement. Auscultation of the chest for breath sounds with ventilation and listening over the stomach for air entry during bagging are helpful. As it is not always possible to visualize the vocal cords in the trauma situation, some people have advocated the addition of an end-tidal CO_2 sensor to the ET tube. If no CO_2 is being produced, the ET tube is in the wrong position. With the initiation of ventilation, rapid increases in the intrathoracic pressure may decrease venous return to the heart, thus precipitating cardiac arrest in the trauma patient with an intravascular volume deficit. Additionally, increased intrathoracic pressure with ventilation increases the size of a pneumothorax and produces a tension pneumothorax. Patients with blunt chest trauma and a closed pneumothorax are at risk. Needle aspiration and placement of a chest tube will rapidly reverse an arrest secondary to a tension pneumothorax. In the trauma situation, it is not unusual to have either penetrating injuries or blunt injuries with an opening from the bronchus into the vascular circulation. Aggressive ventilation may lead to air passage into the circulation which creates air lock in the outflow tract. This may be treated by placing the patient in the left chest up, head down position. If the patient is hemodynamically unstable, this may be impossible. Advancing a central line into the right ventricle and aspirating may eliminate air in the right ventricular outflow tract. Open cardiac massage, aspiration of the ventricle, and aspiration of air from the coronary arteries have all been used to treat this condition. In addition, hyperbaric oxygenation may be of some use in the stable patient. This has been more frequently used for neurologic compromise related to air embolization. Finally, hyperventilation itself creates abnormalities in CO_2 and calcium metabolism which may precipitate an immediate arrest. Hypocapnia can result in systemic vasodilation (although it paradoxically leads to cerebrovascular vasoconstriction) and the acute respiratory alkalosis can cause an acute decrease in the concentration of ionized calcium.

258 A. Blunt iliac artery injury is uncommon because of the protective nature of the bony pelvis. Only 5% of such injuries involve abdominal vessels (the inferior vena cava being the most common). The other 95% involve thoracic vessels. Iliac artery injury is associated with pelvic fracture and with the use of seat belts (rapid deceleration raises an intimal flap causing injury). The diagnosis can be difficult due to lack of clinical symptoms until there is complete occlusion. Only 25% of patients will have markedly diminished pulses and 17% of injuries are diagnosed only after major complications including gross ischemia. Once diagnosed, treatment must include revascularization as the amputation rate with an acutely occluded common iliac artery can approach 50%. Primary repair is usually difficult to perform because of the extensive nature of the flap or destruction of the artery. Reconstruction options include saphenous vein, polytetrafluroethylene (PTFE), or if there has been abdominal contamination, a crossover femor–femoral bypass. Because the rate of associated intra-abdominal injuries exceeds 50% and patients frequently have pelvic fractures, anticoagulation is not appropriate in the acute setting. If there has been prolonged ischemia (more than 4–6 hours), fasciotomy should be considered.

259–261: Questions

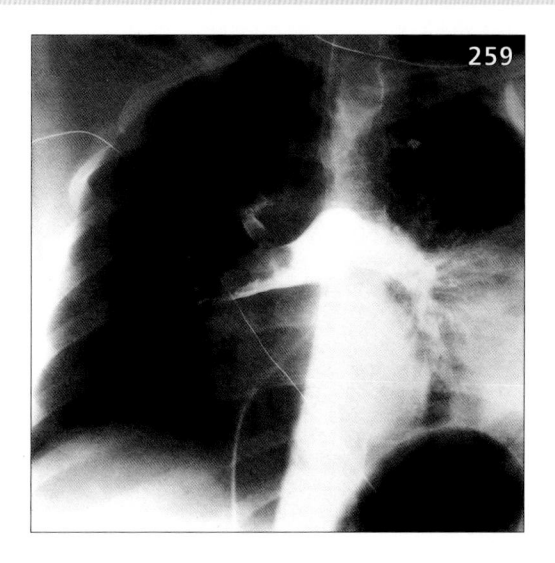

259 A 30-year-old female presents to the emergency room with right-sided chest pain, dyspnea, and hemoptysis. She is noted to have tachypnea and tachycardia. Her chest X-ray is interpreted as normal. She is admitted to the ICU and shortly thereafter has a respiratory arrest. Her BP is 88/50 mmHg (11.7/6.7 kPa), pulse is 134/min, and the blood gas shows a PO_2 of 35 mmHg (4.7 kPa), PCO_2 of 50 mmHg (6.7 kPa), and a pH of 7.30. The patient is intubated, ventilated, and fluid resuscitated with minimal BP response. The PaO_2 on an FiO_2 of 1.0 is 84 mmHg (11.2 kPa), PCO_2 of 36 mmHg (4.8 kPa), and pH of 7.40. The patient is taken to angiography and the pulmonary angiogram is shown (**259**). Discuss the therapeutic options.

260 What is the role of percutaneous transluminal coronary angioplasty relative to thrombolytic therapy in the management of myocardial infarction?

261 Match each drug (A–C) with the effects (1–7):
A Dopamine.
B Dobutamine.
C Amrinone.

1 Increases coronary blood flow.
2 Dose dependent effects.
3 Associated with thrombocytopenia.
4 Peripheral vasoconstrictor.
5 No increase in myocardial O_2 consumption.
6 Increases cAMP.
7 Releases endogenous epinephrine (adrenaline) and norepinephrine (noradrenaline).

259–261: Answers

259 Pulmonary emboli occluding more than 50% of the pulmonary vasculature are associated with acute hemodynamic instability and death. Initial therapy includes the need for systemic heparinization. A large bolus will affect the current clot by inhibiting platelet aggregation and a continuous drip inhibits propagation of the clot by augmenting the action of antithrombin III. Supportive therapy includes maintenance of oxygenation and ventilation using intubation if necessary. Bronchodilators, aminophylline, and corticosteroid may be used to treat the bronchospasm which frequently accompanies pulmonary emboli. Other therapeutic options may include thrombolytic therapy, suction embolectomy, and surgical embolectomy (Trendelenburg procedure). Thrombolytic therapy using streptokinase, urokinase, and t-PA has been trialed. These agents work best on thrombi less than 72 hours old. More rapid lysis of a clot has been documented but the survival advantage has been difficult to show. Transvenous catheter embolectomy is a new modality which supposedly has efficacy similar to surgical embolectomy but with lower morbidity. These claims await verification. Surgical embolectomy is indicated in patients with proven emboli who remain in shock despite exhaustion of other therapies. Published mortality remains near 60%.

260 If it can be performed within 60 minutes of myocardial infarction, primary percutaneous transluminal coronary angioplasty appears to improve patency and clinical outcome when compared to thrombolytic therapy. In patients who present in cardiogenic shock, there is a role for percutaneous transluminal coronary angioplasty in conjunction with percutaneous bypass, analogous to emergency coronary bypass surgery. The role for percutaneous transluminal coronary angioplasty following thrombolytic therapy is limited to patients with evidence of persistent occlusion ('rescue percutaneous transluminal coronary angioplasty') and, or, who have areas of persistent ischemia with a low level stress test following recovery. Routine percutaneous transluminal coronary angioplasty following thrombolytic therapy is discouraged because of the increased complication rates.

261 A and 2, 4, 6; B and 1; C and 3, 5, 6. Dopamine is an endogenous catecholamine which is an immediate precursor of norepinephrine (noradrenaline). It releases both epinephrine (adrenaline) and norepinephrine. The effects of dopamine are dose related. In low doses, it acts on the dopaminergic receptors causing vasodilation. A high dose acts as a vasoconstrictor in the arterial and venous capillary beds. Dobutamine stimulates the $beta_1$-, $beta_2$-, and alpha-receptors. Dobutamine increases myocardial oxygen consumption, but it also increases myocardial oxygen delivery by increasing coronary blood flow as a result of decreased coronary vascular resistance. Amrinone, although a positive inotropic agent, is not related to sympathomimetic stimulation. This drug acts by increasing levels of cAMP and the modulation of intracellular calcium. Amrinone increases cardiac output; however, myocardial oxygenation consumption is not increased. Dose related thrombocytopenia can develop in approximately 3% of patients receiving this medication.

262–264: Questions

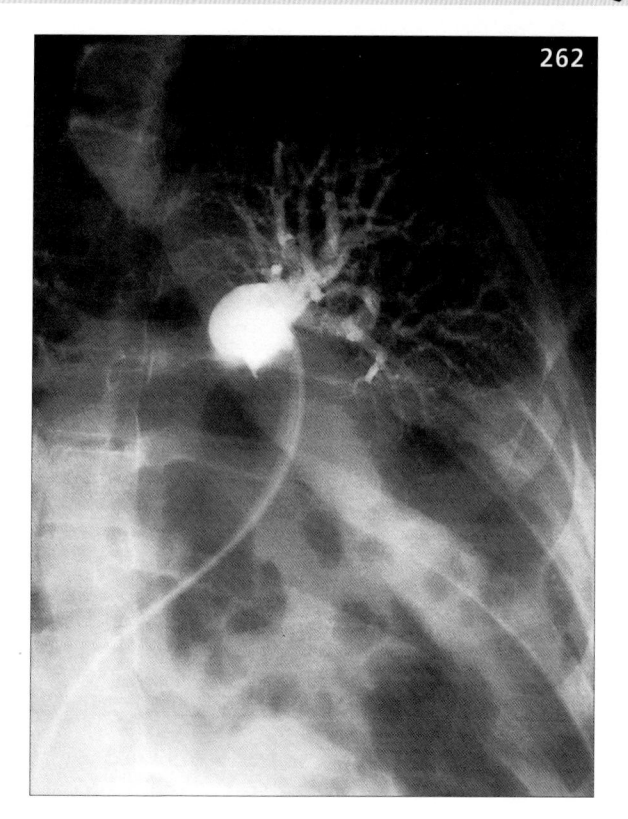

262 This pulmonary angiogram (**262**) was obtained on a 27-year-old male with a closed head injury and a Glasgow coma score of 10. He has a left acetabular fracture with an open compound fracture on the left tibia with extensive tissue loss. There is also a right femoral neck fracture. The patient requires several more orthopedic procedures. What therapy would you advise?

263 A 20-year-old patient injured in a motor vehicle accident had a laparotomy with suture repair of his liver fracture. He has a closed suction drain placed in Morrison's pouch and a penrose drain placed over a contused area of the pancreas. He develops profuse drainage from the penrose drain site. How will you evaluate this?

264 Discuss briefly the management of vasospasm following subarachnoid hemorrhage.

262–264: Answers

262 This pulmonary embolus probably came from the pelvic veins. As he requires more orthopedic procedures, he is at risk for other pulmonary emboli. In view of his injuries from trauma which would include the closed head injury and the orthopedic injuries, he is at risk for bleeding from therapy with lytic agents (t-PA, streptokinase) so that this is contraindicated. Heparinizing this patient increases his risk of pelvic bleeding and intracranial hemorrhage with worsening of his neurologic status. A vena cava filter should be placed in this patient which would decrease the pulmonary effects of recurrent emboli. The patient should have careful cardiorespiratory monitoring. Consultation with the neurosurgeon will assist in the timing of heparin therapy if necessary.

263 The drainage should be collected and quantified, and the electrolytes, bilirubin, and amylase content should be measured. The fluid analysis identifies the injured organ. This patient could have either a biliary or pancreatic fistula. The chart lists the electrolyte content of pancreatic fluid and bile (in mmol/l, mEq/l).

Secretion	Na^+	K^+	Cl^-	HCO_3^-
Pancreatic	135–155	4–6	60–110	70–90
Bile	135–155	4–6	80–110	35–50

Pancreatic fluid contains amylase and bile contains bilirubin. The amylase is elevated in this drainage. Conservative therapy is generally applied with the use of intravenous fluid and electrolyte replacement, and total parenteral nutrition. Somatostatin is given in an attempt to close the fistula. Imaging techniques such as a CT scan or endoscopic retrograde cholangiopancreatography may be helpful to identify the area of leakage. If the pancreatic fistula does not close with conservative therapy, surgical intervention with either pancreatic resection or Roux-en-y reconstruction is performed.

264 Vasospasm appears to be mediated by the presence of RBCs in the subarachnoid space, is greater with aneurysmal subarachnoid hemorrhage than nonaneurysmal subarachnoid hemorrhage, and may involve mediation by local vasoactive agents such as endothelin-1. The risk correlated with the amount of blood in the subarachnoid space, is increased if glucose is >6.7 mmol/l (120 mg/dl) in the first week and possibly by the use of e-aminocaproic acid to prevent rebleeding. Prophylaxis includes hypertensive therapy (to ensure a pulmonary capillary wedge pressure of <18 mmHg (2.4 kPa) as patients are at increased risk of pulmonary edema), calcium channel blockers (nimodipine), vasopressors, and occasionally hemodilution (hemoglobin 100–110 g/l [10–11 g/dl]). Diagnosis of vasospasm is usually clinical, the commonest general symptom being simply a decreased active interaction of the patient with family/nursing staff. Transcranial Doppler (TCD) may reveal elevated flow (velocities >120 cm/sec) but appear to often underestimate the incidence and severity of vasospasm. Once vasospasm is occurring, treatment includes the above mentioned hypertensive therapy, antivasospastic therapy, and occasionally interventional methods with papavarine or angioplasty.

265–268: Questions

265 Give the differential diagnosis for the effusion drained in the photograph (**265**).

266 What are the class 1 antidysrhythmics?

267 A 72-year-old male was brought to the emergency department because he was confused and had some seizure activity. An initial laboratory work-up reveals a sodium level of 115 mmol/l (mEq/l), but is otherwise normal. His chest X-ray demonstrates a new lung lesion. What is the management and the diagnosis?

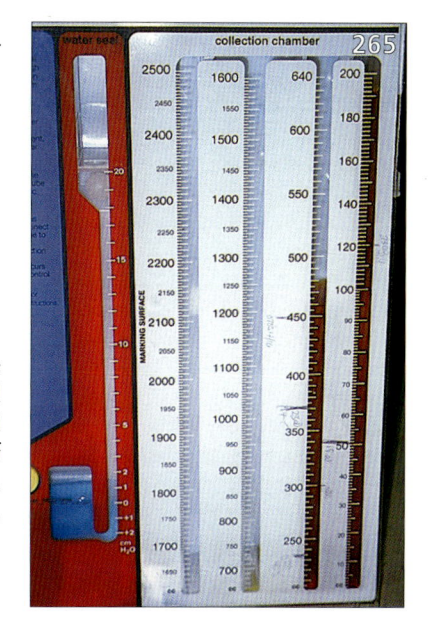

268 A 25-year-old female weighing 58 kg (128 lb) became septic after undergoing a colon resection with primary anastomosis for ulcerative colitis. Triple antibiotics were instituted. At 0900 hours the hemodynamic parameters shown below are obtained. The patient's abdomen is distended and tympanitic with no obvious evidence of peritoneal signs. On the basis of this hemodynamic profile, what is your next step?
A Administer steroids.
B Administer blood.
C Administer Ringer's lactate.
D Renal dose dopamine 3 µg/kg/min.
E Dobutamine 5 µg/kg/min.

Input measured	DO_2 989 ml/min	PAWP 15 mmHg (2.0 kPa)
CO 6.76 l/min	DO_2I 611 ml/min/m²	CVP 13 mmHg (1.7 kPa)
FiO_2 0.3	VO_2 185 ml/min	
PaO_2 104 mmHg (13.9 kPa)	VO_2I 114 ml/min/m²	Hemodynamics
$PaCO_2$ 31 mmHg (4.1 kPa)	Aa grad 73 mmHg (9.7 kPa)	output/derived
PvO_2 40 mmHg (5.3 kPa)	Qs/Qt 23%	CI 4.17 l/min/m²
Hgb 108 g/l (10.8 g/dl)		SV 73 ml/b
Pbar 760 mmHg	Hemodynamics	EDV 169 ml
(101.3 kPa)	input/measured	EDVI 104.4 ml/m²
	CO 6.76 l/min	SVR 958 dyn.sec/cm⁵
Output derived	HR 93/min	SVRI 1,552 dyn.sec/cm⁵/m²
CaO_2 14.63 ml/dl	REF 43	PVR 95 dyn.sec/cm⁵
CvO_2 11.9 ml/dl	MAP 94 mmHg (12.5 kPa)	PVRI 153 dyn.sec/cm⁵/m²
$AVDO_2$ 2.73 ml/dl	MPAP 23 mmHg (3.1 kPa)	

265–268: Answers

265 Bloody effusions are most commonly caused by trauma, malignancy, and tuberculosis. Blunt or penetrating trauma may cause this clinical picture and be associated with rib fractures and pulmonary contusions. Surgery on the heart, lungs, esophagus, chest wall, diaphragm, or intra-abdominal organs may result in sanguinous drainage. Any tumor may seed the pleural space but the most common are lung, breast, ovarian, and gastric. Primary mesothelioma may also result in bloody effusions. Tuberculosis is more likely to give this appearance than are other infections.

266 Class 1, the local anesthetics, have been divided into three subsets. *Class 1A* includes quinidine, procainamide, and dysopyramide. All three can be used for supra-ventricular as well as ventricular dysrhythmias. All three can prolong the Q–T interval and induce Torsades. They should not be given for wide complex tachyarrhythmias, therefore, unless one is sure that the arrhythmia is not ventricular. If the length of QRS increases more than 50%, procainamide should be withheld. Side effects include hypotension, drowsiness, myalgia, and Raynauds. Both procainamide and quinidine are useful in treating supraventricular and ventricular arrhythmias. Quinidine results in increased digoxin levels, necessitating adjustment of dosing. It should be noted that as a rule, drug levels of both quinidine and procainamide/N-acycle procainamide do not appear to correlate well with efficacy or predicting complications. *Class 1B* agents include lidocaine, phenytoin, tocainamide, and mexiletine. These agents have little effect on atrial dysrhythmias. Lidocaine is associated with proarrhythmic effects, myocardial depression, and CNS side effects including seizures. The incidence of side effects is greater in the presence of CHF. Phenytoin is used only to treat digoxin induced arrhythmias. Infusion rates should be <50 mg/min to avoid cardiovascular collapse. *Class 1C* agents include flecainide and encainide. These agents were tried in a study of long-term suppression of ventricular ectopy following myocardial infarction. Proarrhythmic rates of up to 25% were noted with possibly increased mortality. These agents are restricted to resistant malignant ventricular tachyarrhythmias.

267 Lung cancers can be associated with a variety of nonmetastatic extrathoracic symptoms including the syndrome of inappropriate antidiuretic hormone. This is particularly associated with small cell lung cancer. The diagnosis is made by a low sodium and a low serum osmolality in the face of an inappropriately elevated urine concentration and urine sodium levels. The primary therapy for the syndrome of inappropriate antidiuretic hormone is directed against the underlying lesion and includes possibly surgical resection, radiation, or chemotherapy. Management of the hyponatremia includes water restriction and the careful use of 3% sodium chloride. An overly rapid correction of the hypernatremia, however, can lead to central pontine myelinolysis and should be avoided.

268 C. This patient is volumed depleted and vasodilated secondary to sepsis, VO_2 and VO_2I are low due to peripheral shunting. The filling pressures, although normal, are low for this patient. SVRI is high due to a high MAP and low CVP.

269, 270: Questions

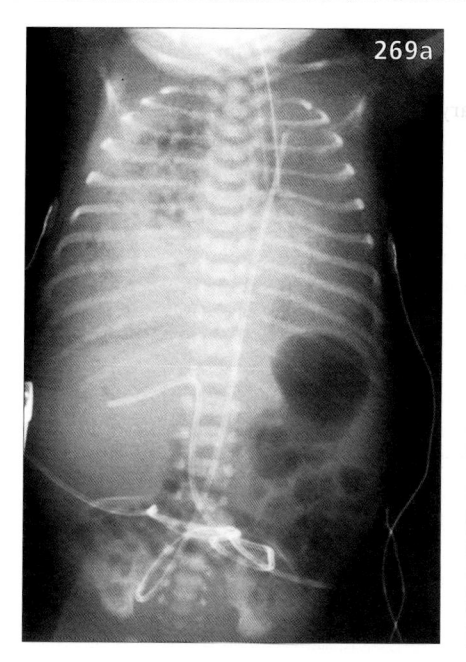

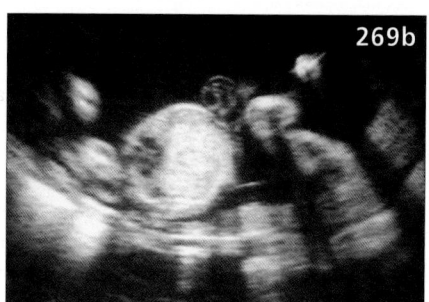

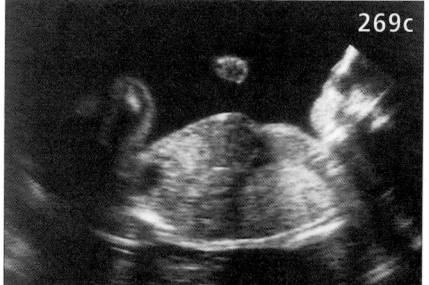

269 A newborn infant male weighing 1.6 kg (3 lb 8 oz) is diagnosed *in utero* with a space occupying lesion in the right thoracic cavity (**269a–d**). His twin is normal on ultrasound. He is delivered at 32 weeks gestation and is tachypneic and hypoxic requiring intubation and conventional ventilation with a FiO_2 of 0.75.

Management of this infant would ideally be which of the following?
A Immediate arterial venous (or veno–venous) cannulation and placement on ECMO.
B Administration of surfactant.
C Selective endobronchial intubation and ventilation.
D Thoracotomy and lobectomy.
E High frequency oscillatory ventilation.

270 What factors contribute to heparin resistance?

269, 270: Answers

269 B and D. The chest X-ray shows a classic picture of a cystic adenomatoid malformation–mixture of solid and cystic elements with mediastinal shift. In addition the child is premature and there are changes consistent with hyaline membrane disease. The *in utero* ultrasound shows a solid space occupying lesion in the chest. ECMO is not indicated in this child for a number of reasons. He is too small for successful cannulation and ECMO, but more importantly the usual other conventional means of ventilatory support have not been used. Ideally, administration of surfactant would be the first line of treatment, to help correct the hyaline membrane disease, along with conventional ventilation. Once the child is stabilized, removal of the space occupying lesion in the right chest via thoracotomy and lobectomy represents the ideal treatment. The appearance in the chest X-ray may be confused with a congenital diaphramgatic hernia but there is no apparent herniation of abdominal viscera and the appearance suggests that both diaphragms are intact. The mediastinal shift and atelectasis are the primary cause of respiratory problems but very rarely one sees persistent pulmonary hypertension which may ultimately necessitate the use of nitric oxide and subsequently ECMO (in an appropriately sized child).

270 Heparin resistance is defined as a requirement for >35,000 IU of heparin every 24 hours. The anticoagulant effect of heparin is modified by platelet, fibrin, vascular surfaces, and plasma proteins. Platelets bind factor Xa protecting it from inactivation by the heparin–antithrombin III complex. Platelets also secrete platelet factor 4, a protein which neutralizes heparin. Heparin-induced thrombocytopenia does not become manifest until 7–10 days after treatment initiation. The destroyed platelets may release platelet factor 4, neutralizing heparin's anticoagulant activity. Fibrin binds thrombin protecting it from inactivation by heparin. This contributes to the higher concentrations of heparin required to prevent formation of venous thromboses. Certain proteins elevated in inflammatory or malignant disorders can bind heparin, neutralizing its anticoagulant activity. Numerous drugs are thought to interfere with the anticoagulant effect of heparin. Some of these may cause artifactual resistance, by altering partial thromboplastin time (PTT) levels. Acute phases reactants including factor VIII and fibrinogen, can shorten the PTT, falsely suggesting heparin resistance. Heparin assays will allow artifactual resistance to be distinguished from physiologic resistance. A continuous stimulus for low-grade activation of the clotting cascade (e.g. disseminated intravascular coagulation) can result in heparin resistance by consumption of antithrombin III and release of platelet factor 4. Preoperative heparin can lead to intraoperative heparin resistance, thought secondary to large increases in platelet factor 4 after intraoperative administration. Continuous heparin use may deplete antithrombin III, reducing subsequent effectiveness of heparin. Heparin resistance is also seen with intra-aortic balloon support, oral contraceptive use, recent thrombolytics, pregnancy, and increased platelet levels. Direct assays of heparin levels should be performed when heparin resistance is suspected.

271, 272: Questions

271 A 60-year-old male, a life-long smoker, has had daily productive sputum for the past 2 years.
i. What is the life-threatening condition apparent on this X-ray (**271a**)?
ii. He needs to be ventilated due to exhaustion, what ventilatory options are available?
iii. How would you set a ventilator if endotracheal intubation has already occurred?

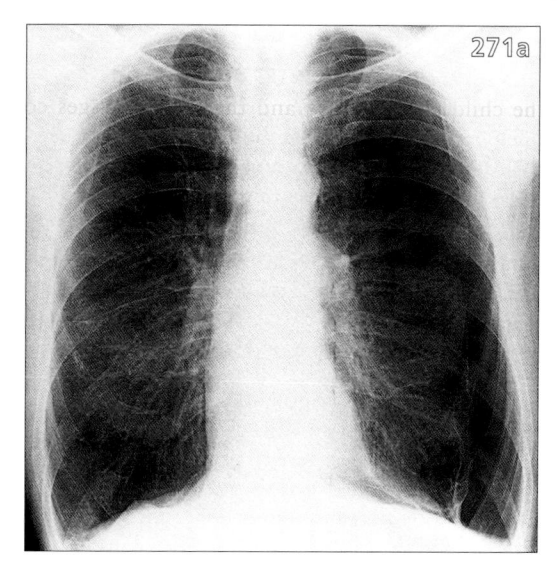

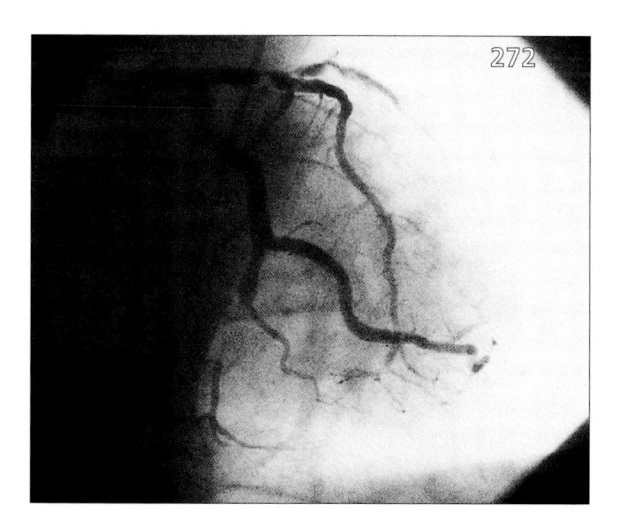

272 A 47-year-old female is admitted for an elective angioplasty of a proximal LAD/diagonal stenosis (**272**). After ballooning each lesion successively using a two-wire technique, the patient develops crushing chest pain just as she is being transferred to the stretcher to leave the catheter laboratory.
i. Discuss the further management of this patient, with attention to indications for surgical intervention following acute angioplasty failure.
ii. Discuss pertinent operative details in this patient.

189

271, 272: Answers

271 i. This patient has an acute exacerbation of COPD. This is manifest by the obvious increased lung markings throughout both lung fields. His condition is complicated by a large simple pneumothorax (**271b**, arrowed). This could easily become a tension pneumothorax if the patient's lungs are subjected to positive pressure ventilation. A chest drain must be inserted as soon as possible. If the patient is 'in extremis' then urgent intubation can occur and a wide-bore IV cannula is placed in the 2nd intercostal space midclavicular line as a stop gap measure to prevent the pneumothorax from 'tensioning'.

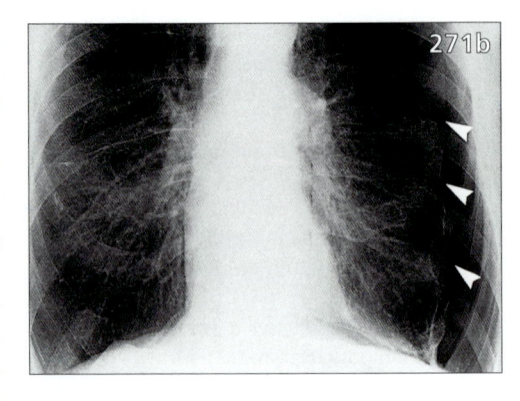

ii. Two options are open to manage this patient depending on whether the patient is exhausted or not. Intubation may not be necessary. Non-invasive positive pressure ventilation may be possible. In true exhaustion, however, a skilled anesthesiologist or emergency room physician should electively intubate the patient. BP usually drops precipitously with a combination of positive pressure ventilation and induction of anesthesia. Great care is needed in selection of suitability and dose of induction agents. Fluids and pressor agents should be available to counter this expected BP drop.

iii. Ventilator settings are difficult to judge in a patient like this. Airway pressures can be very high but equally the patient needs an adequate minute volume to achieve gas exchange. It is best to limit the upper airway pressure to no more than 35–40 cmH$_2$O. Aiming for tidal volumes of 10 ml/kg is probably reasonable to start with but observation of the airway pressure and chest wall movements is vital. It is likely that the lungs will be noncompliant and therefore some degree of 'underventilation' is likely to prevent further pneumothoraces. Hypercapnia can be tolerated (up to 52.5 mmHg (7.0 kPa)) until the exacerbation (and possible septic sequelae) is treated. Good bronchial toilet, beta agonists (salbutamol/albuterol) and physiotherapy will assist in keeping airway pressures low.

272 i. Initial treatment usually involves further angioplastic interventions, or some method to provide temporary distal flow, such as a perfusion catheter. If cardiogenic shock is a feature, intra-aortic balloon pumping will be of benefit. Definitive treatment is expeditious coronary artery bypass grafting, if the vessel cannot be reopened.

ii. The operative approach is based upon the degree of ischemia, the hemodynamic stability, underlying ventricular function, comorbidity, and the patient's age. Severe, prolonged ischemia necessitates immediate institution of cardiopulmonary bypass. Although the internal mammary may be taken down, this is inadvisable in the very elderly, those with severe comorbidity, cardiogenic shock, or severe pre-existing ventricular dysfunction, in whom vein grafts should be employed. Cardioplegia may be delivered antegrade successfully, but there is a theoretical benefit to retrograde delivery when coronary occlusions are present.

Index

All references are to question and answer numbers

Abdominal radiology 172
Acetaminopen overdose 2
Acid-base imbalance 19, 27, 202
Adrenergic receptors 190
Airway compromise 4, 93, 97
Amniotic fluid embolism 41
Amrinone 122, 261
Amylase, serum 101
Anaphylaxis 21, 174, 235
Anesthesia 113, 118
Anticoagulant agents 195
Antidiuretic hormone, syndrome of inappropriate 267
Antidotes 239
Antidysrhythmics 46, 124, 143, 266
Antimicrobial agents 84
Antithrombin III deficiency 38
Aortic aneurysm, abdominal 82, 91, 242, 247
Aortic stenosis 148
Aortic/great vessel injury 105
Appendicitis 52
ARDS 140, 192
Arterial catheters 218, 256
Asthma, acute 40, 126, 203
$AVDO_2$ 5, 227

Bacterial translocation 224
Biliary leak 9
Bleeding, hidden 249
Blood gases 27, 223
Blue toe syndrome 194
Bronchoesophageal fistula, congenital 57
Bronchoscopy 17
Bronchospasm 26, 253
Burn wounds 50, 74, 103, 156, 197, 234

Calcium antagonists 124
Candida albicans 196
Carbon dioxide monitoring 12, 133, 207, 231
Carbon monoxide poisoning 108
Cardiac arrest 186, 207, 257
Cardiac dysrhythmias 29, 225
Cardiac output 56
Cardiac tamponade 51, 149
Cerebrovascular disease 13, 191, 193, 246, 264
Cervial spine pathology 97
Chemotherapy 80, 232
Cholecystectomy, laparoscopic 9
Cholecystitis, acalculous 139, 209
Chylous fistula 39
Clostridium difficile 81, 167
Clostridium perfringens 114
Colitis, ischemic 1

pseudomembranous 55
Colonic pseudo-obstruction, acute 45
Compartment syndromes 87, 179, 219
COPD 113, 271
Coronary artery bypass grafting 85, 272
Coronary artery disease 191
CPR 128, 231
Creatinine clearance 33, 229
Cystic adenomatoid malformation 269

Deadspace disease 125
Deep vein thrombosis 31
Diabetic ketoacidosis 187
Diaphragmatic herniae, congenital 65
Diaphragmatic injury 64, 138, 230
Diarrhea 81, 167
Dieulafoy 'ulcers' 61
Digoxin toxicity 88
Diuretics 86, 162
Dobutamine 122, 233, 261
Dopamine 122, 261
Duodenal ulcers 130

ECMO 23, 163
Electrical injuries 90, 164
Emphysema, bullous 211
  congenital lobar 8
Enalapril 208
Endocarditis, tricuspid 181
Epiglottitis 93, 120
Epinephrine 21, 122, 233
Erysipelas 4
Escharotomy, chest wall 156
Escherichia coli 95, 111
Esmolol 208, 233
Esophageal perforation, benign 170
Esophageal varices 215, 228

Febrile neutropenia 232
Fetal circulation, persistent 23
Fluid balance 28, 59, 159, 197
Foreign body 17
Fractures 137, 169, 219, 262

Gallstones 110, 112, 115
Gastric fistula 123
Gastric ulcer 254
Glasgow coma score 106
Global cerebral hypoxemia-ischemia injury 132

Haemophilus influenzae 92, 95
Head injury 106, 262
Heart block 107
Hematochezia 201
Hemodialysis 210
Hemothorax 146
Heparin resistance 270

191

Index

Hepatitis, exposure risk 168
HIV/AIDS 15, 16, 52, 160, 168
Hydralazine 208
Hydrochloric acid injury 244
Hydrofluoric acid burns 213
Hypermagnesemia 212
Hyperthermia, malignant 3, 129
Hypothermia 75

Ileostomy 73
Iliac artery injury 258
Incidence 14
Inhalation agents 10, 93, 109, 226
Inhalation injury 108, 200
Intestinal ischemia 1, 79, 242
Intubation, difficulties 6, 97
Ion channels, cardiac muscle cells 222
Isuprel 122
IV fat emulsions 53

Klebsiella pneumoniae 95, 135

Legionella pneumophila 7, 95
Line sepsis 238
Liver injury 11, 105, 173, 263
Lung abscess 251
Lung collapse 27, 142

Mallory–Weiss tears 188
Marasmus malnutrition 144
Meningitis 63
Mesenteric ischemia, non-occlusive 248
Mesenteric thrombosis 161
Microcirculatory thrombosis 189
Myocardial cell physiology 220, 250
Myocardial infarction 116, 241, 243, 247, 260
Myocardial ischemia, acute 184
Myoglobinuria 137

Nasoenteric tube 34, 147
Necrotizing soft tissue infections 165, 180, 185
Neisseria meningitidis 63, 95
Nitric oxide 204
Nitroprusside 208, 233
NonHodgkin lymphoma 22

Organophosphate insecticides 102

Pancreatic injury 101, 263
Pancreatitis 47, 53, 110, 175, 236
Paracentesis catheter 134
Paraesophageal hernia 34, 36
Percutaneous transluminal coronary angioplasty 260
Perineal gangrene 66
Peritoneal lavage 153
Placenta previa 30
Pleural effusions 131, 265

Pneumobilia 60
Pneumothorax 25, 147, 151, 183, 245
Poisoning 102, 108, 239
Portal hypertension 228
Postpartum hemorrhage 30, 176
Pre-eclampsia 35
Pregnancy 35, 41, 118, 128
Prevalence 14
Pseudoaneurysm, femoral artery 42
Pseudomonas aeruginosa 50, 95
Psoriasis 15, 16
Pulmonary artery catheterization 70, 76, 156, 157, 198
Pulmonary capillary wedge pressure 20, 122
Pulmonary embolism 31, 67, 128, 133, 176, 259, 262
Pulse oximetry 74

Refeeding syndrome 150
Renal function 33, 54, 99, 100, 212, 229
Resting energy expenditure 62
Right ventricular infarction 171

Shock 44, 58, 235, 252
Sickle cell disease 71
Small bowel injury 240
Soft-tissue infections 94, 165, 180, 185
Splenic injury 119
Staphylococcus aureus 121
Status epilepticus 78, 96, 98, 109, 155, 217
Streptococcus pneumoniae 43, 71
Subarachnoid hemorrhage 13, 246, 264
SVO_2 182
Swan–Ganz catheter 20, 56
Systemic inflammatory response syndrome 58
Systemic vascular resistance 166

Thoracostomy drainage system 152
Thoracotomy, resuscitative 186
Thrombocytopenia 221
Thrombolytic therapy 184, 195, 241, 260
Total parenteral nutrition 24, 48, 150, 237, 238
Tracheobronchogial injury 72
Tracheoesophageal fistula 206
Tracheoinnominate fistula 255
Tracheostomy 151, 214, 255
Tricyclic antidepressants 69
Tumor lysis syndrome 37

Urinalysis 33, 54, 137, 229
Urine output 99

Vascular reconstruction 145
Ventilation 18, 32, 68, 127, 136, 141, 154, 156, 177, 178
Ventricular septal rupture 117

Wounds 89, 138, 145, 149, 216